MW00988626

Seven Days in Usha Village:

A Conversation with

Dr. Sebi

Copyright © 2007

Beverly Oliver

ALL RIGHTS RESERVED. No part of this book may be reproduced or transmitted in any form or by any means, electronic or mechanical, including photocopying, recording, or by any information storage and retrieval system, without permission in writing from the publisher. Brief quotations may be used in literary reviews.

Cover Design by Robert Porter

ISBN: 978-0-615-18681-8

Published by Dr. Sebi's Office, Inc.

ACKNOWLEDGMENTS

An adaptation of John Donne's *Meditation 17* says "No man is an island, no man stands alone." And with that in mind I thank the following individuals for their cooperation, creativity and editorial expertise: Robert Porter, Steve Jones, Wanda Thomas and Michael Barto. Xave Bowman and Nina Taylor-Collins assured an unbroken line of communication at Dr. Sebi's Office, Inc. and I'm most grateful for the connection. And of course I give many thanks to the source, the green light for this book, Dr. Sebi and his wife Matun (Patricia Bowman), whose generosity and dedication to healing remain impeccable. To the Creator of our vast, wonderful Universe thank you, thank you, a thousand times thank you for this Journey.

CONTENTS

INTRODUCTION

I met him in Washington, DC in the early 1980s when I produced public affairs features for WHUR-FM, and shortly after his transition from Alfredo Bowman the steam engineer to Dr. Sebi the herbalist. My own gynecological concerns were an issue at the time and I shared my feelings with colleagues at the station. One in particular, an engineer and vegetarian named John Davies, suggested I meet a man who might remedy my problems. I decided to see him instead of having a laparoscopy.

When I saw him for the first time at the Community Warehouse in DC, Dr. Sebi stood tall, slender, statuesque, much like a Maasai tribesman in East Africa. When he spoke, English words flowed clearly and robustly from his Yul Brynner-sounding voice even though his first language is Spanish. And his persona, as I recall, resembled Mr. Brynner's character, the King of Siam, in the film *The King and I.*

Words about natural and unnatural foods and his analogies of human and animal physiology, especially gorillas and polar bears, pulsated throughout the room. No microphone or bull horn needed. Some listeners sat surprised by his lecture, interjecting soft murmurs of doubt. Others willingly and intently received the message. I was one of them, and because I felt an even larger audience should hear Dr. Sebi's perspective on health and nutrition, I invited him to WHUR to speak in a four-part radio series on herbs and natural healing. He came.

We recorded a session a little over an hour and as I think back, it was a difficult edit. You just can't put it all in the program, no matter how great or informative. The final cut yielded four 10-minute shows with theme music by Lonnie Liston Smith. WHUR broadcast the series in the newsmagazine *The Sunday Digest.*

Subsequently, throughout the mid-80s I traveled to New York City to hear Dr. Sebi's lectures. After that period my career path changed somewhat, taking me out of the East Coast. The New York Attorney General's office attempted to change Dr. Sebi's in 1987 when it arrested and jailed him for refusing to remove unlicensed medical claims from New York City newspapers *The Amsterdam News* and *The Village Voice.* His advertisements promoted cures for AIDS, asthma, cancer, and sickle cell anemia. He won his case in 1988, continued to treat clients with his products, but would eventually relocate his office. Twenty years would pass before Dr. Sebi and I reconnected. That happened in 2005 in Los Angeles, California, two years after I moved to the West Coast to continue my career as a writer and creative artist.

In our first conversation since reconnecting I asked him why he hadn't written about his knowledge of health and nutrition. Lo and behold he pulled out a manuscript, a draft of his autobiography. Words cannot fully explain how I felt that moment. Such a thrill to know the public can now have a reference book of more than 25 years experience in nutrition and natural healing from Dr. Sebi's perspective and experiences.

I was equally moved when asked to assist with his work-in-progress, thus, the reason for the seven-day interview in Usha Village and La Ceiba, Honduras November 6-12, 2005. Reading this book, *Seven Days in Usha Village: A Conversation with Dr. Sebi,* you experience part of that sojourn.

Mountains filled with lush, dark green tropical trees and plants surround Dr. Sebi's Usha Village, a healing center in a town called Agua Caliente, 24 miles east of La Ceiba. His thermal hot spring runs from the mountains straight down to the middle of his 14 cabins—he calls them huts. An African mask hangs over the yellow hut once occupied by the late hip hop singer

Lisa "Left Eye" Lopes. Like others before her, she sought healing and contemplation at Usha Village.

Several mornings I stepped outside my cabin and experienced a natural pedicure as warm waters from the hot spring flowed over my bare feet. I usually use a cream moisturizer on my feet after bathing. No need for that at the village.

The hot spring is also the source for Dr. Sebi's sauna and bath houses. One of its healing properties is the existence of sulfur *(p. 67)*, beneficial in treating AIDS and lung cancer.

Never in my life have I known a man so passionate about herbs and plants that he'll stop driving a vehicle to go check out one seen from his windshield. He risked going to jail for his curiosity about a plant he saw on private property in Brazil *(pp. 85-86)*. That's what I learned about Dr. Sebi while tape recording the interview and riding around the town of La Ceiba in the back seat of his truck, his wife Matun seated in front.

Speaking of a love affair with plants, I'm the offspring of Southern parents (South Carolina). Imagine my reaction when Dr. Sebi gives the thumbs down to collard greens, a plant I've eaten since time immemorial *(p. 82)*.

Over the past 20 years Dr. Sebi has advised and treated many celebrities and community activists. Some experiences proved invaluable to all involved. Others stirred intense emotions that resurfaced during the seven-day interview *(pp. 98, 111)*. His mother Violet, who recently passed at age 92, also witnessed her son's heated energy *(p. 112)*. But note Dr. Sebi's love for one of the most prominent influences in his life, his grandmother Mama Hay, for whom his autobiography is named *(p. 12)*.

Intense? Yes. Unconventional? Undoubtedly, yet Dr. Sebi's generosity remains unquestionable. Evidence of that is in your hands. *Seven Days in Usha Village: A*

Conversation with Dr. Sebi precedes Dr. Sebi's autobiography, a project started long before this publication. He agreed to go forward with this book to commemorate the 20th anniversary of winning his court case, and as a means of informing his supporters his autobiography is on the way. Dr. Sebi generously allowed excerpts from *The Cure: The Autobiography of Dr. Sebi "Mama Hay"* to be printed here. You'll read italicized passages from the autobiography that relate to topics discussed in the interview. In a way one book supports the other.

—Beverly Oliver

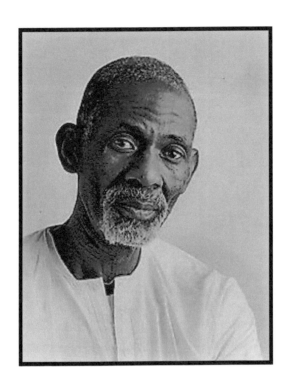

**Alfredo Bowman
(Dr. Sebi)**

PROLOGUE

Approximately 45 years ago I made the statement "I want to be useful. I want to do something great for the Black woman so the world can see how amazing, how beautiful she is." I remember sitting in a barber's chair in New Orleans in 1960 when I made that statement. I was bent on giving her something that would elevate her universally. It was a drive that I could not contain. It came from within—an inner dictate. I didn't know that I would have to face the American Medical Association, the Food and Drug Administration and the judicial system of the State of New York in representing the gift that I was going to give her, the Black Woman of the world.

—The Cure: The Autobiography of Dr. Sebi "Mama Hay"

~~~~~~~~~~~~~~~~~~~~~~~~~~~~~~

Mama Hay—Beginnings

~~~~~~~~~~~~~~~~~~~~~~~~~~~~~~

Mama Hay—Beginnings

Dr. Sebi: Well, hey, me, I'm out the bush. Dr. Sebi was born and grew up in the bush. So the dictates that provided me the environment that I have internally and mentally is not the same as a child born and grew up in a city. I grew up, I saw snakes. I could tell you the different snakes, spiders, bush, the herbs, the taste of them, the birds, because I grew up in that.

Beverly: Were you experimenting with herbs then?

Dr. Sebi: No, no, no. I just knew the herb. Most Hondurans know herbs. Most young boys and girls from the Caribbean know herbs. They know herbs.

Beverly: What about the healing?

Dr. Sebi: They may not know about the healing properties of the herbs but they know herbs. And I knew that herb. I didn't even know the healing properties until recently.

I remember my life distinctly from age three because I had an experience that I will never forget. I was playing by the Aguan River and did not realize that the water was too deep.

Dr. Sebi: What happened is I went to the river and the river wasn't too far from the house and I saw this shrimp. And the shrimp was huge to me but I know it was something I wasn't supposed to take out of the water. And the shrimp kept backing up, and kept backing up deeper, deeper into the river and I was following the shrimp. When I looked, I was in a hole. And I was holding on to these logs and these logs were turning over and wouldn't let me grip them.

---

* All italicized paragraphs—excerpts from the manuscript *The Cure: The Autobiography of Dr. Sebi "Mama Hay."*

I had to hold onto logs and float to shore. I ran all the way home dripping wet. My mother never knew that before I arrived that day I had been fighting for my life in the river. That was the first indication of the importance of water in my life.

Beverly: Who is Mama Hay?

Dr. Sebi: Mama Hay is a young lady that was born in Belize. She was born in the Protectorate, the Principality of Belize under the British at the time. About her life with her mother, I know very little. I know a lot about her life with her grandmother, which was Elizabeth. Elizabeth was my grandmother's grandmother. And according to my grandmother she was a very tall woman, very strong woman. She lived until the age of 124. Then my grandmother, Mama Hay, was born to Carolina. Carolina had two girls. Mama Hay was one. I don't remember the name of the other girl. Mama Hay grew up very attached to her mother. Mama Hay never even had a boyfriend until she was already age 28. And a young man who was very much in love with her came to, you know, ask her to be his mate. But Mama Hay said no. She didn't feel good with the man. And as my grandmother telling me the story, I could look into her eyes and tell that when a woman doesn't want a man, it's not that she doesn't want him because he's lesser than another. She just doesn't feel right with him. She doesn't resonate with him. She said no, no, no, no many times. Well, one night the man in question came and shot my grandmother in her left breast towards her heart. They took my grandmother to the hospital thinking that she would be dead. Everybody thought she would die. But my grandmother lived. And then she said I think I can leave Belize now. I should leave Belize. She left Belize and she came to Honduras. She came to Honduras in the year of 1914 and she met this man that took her off her heels. His name was Ben Francis. He

6

was a Haitian. This Haitian gave my grandmother love and a life that even when she was telling me the story, and she was already in her 70s, 80s, the laughter, the love that this man brought to her was still showing in her face. He was from Haiti and she bore him two children, Violet and Lucius. Lucius left very early for the United States. Violet stayed and took care of Mama Hay until she passed. Mama Hay wasn't a woman that you invite to a dance. She was never part of any sorority. She was never part of a lodge. She was never part of anything. She was never invited to anything. Mama Hay was a very secluded lady, very, very, very private. And I didn't notice that I would be going to sleep every night at 6 o'clock. And it was because of Mama Hay. Mama Hay would tell me these stories because Mama Hay took possession of me when I was 8 and she took care of me until I was about 11.

Beverly: Why did Mama Hay take possession of you at the age of 8?

Dr. Sebi: Because she had met another man by the name of Duncan from Jamaica.

Beverly: Your grandmother?

Dr. Sebi: My mother met another man from Jamaica named Duncan after my father was killed. My father was killed.

Beverly: Do you know how or why?

Dr. Sebi: Yes, I know how and why and I even met the man that killed him. I met the man in New Orleans. His name was Earl Bellcarris. They called him Monterey "the hand of a tiger." He killed my father, paid by people to kill him to come into possession of the land of my grandfather. And I have the papers in my hand right

7

now. All the land of my grandfather is my possession. But my father was killed because of that. But my father also was a very angry man. He used to look for trouble.

Beverly: What was his name?

Dr. Sebi: His name was Clifford, Clifford Bowman. A man came to me once and said that the gun that he showed me was the gun that he bought to kill my father with. So Mama Hay had me under her tutelage in whatever from age 8. At age 11, I became a caddie and then I went to work in the Miramar Standard Fruit Company, dairy farm. It was called Miramar. I worked until I was 14. Then I left Miramar and went to work in the commissary. And Mama Hay became even closer because I would work hours that gave me more hours with her. In listening to her I learned from my grandmother that the thing she prized more than all is her independence. Her independence. It was easy for her to leave Belize. It was easy for her to tell the man that shot her she didn't love him. Some women would have played it off in a way to not hurt the individual. Not my grandmother. She was straight up front. She didn't like this man and she was shot because of it. So Mama Hay suffered at the hands of the Black man, her brother, what is still continuing to perpetuate. The Black man, many of us are very abusive and rightfully so, because the very food that precipitates the abuse is being fed to us by our wives. So you see, it's a vicious cycle. Mama Hay made sure that I did not become an alcoholic. She made sure that the need for anything was zero. Whether I had a girlfriend or not, it didn't mean anything to Mama Hay. Mama Hay told me at 7 years of age that I didn't need a duck for a birthday present, that I didn't need anything or anyone. So Mama Hay, in reality, is the pillar of my foundation. She is the very pillar in which all of the things that I have done lays on Mama Hay, because of her instilling in me the attitude of doing, not

8

talking. My grandmother was a doer. She was a woman that didn't go to the school but she provided a life for herself in Honduras, when it was most difficult. Yes she did. And she gave her grandson certain ethical and moral standards because she knew that one day I would have to face the world. So she felt she had to give me this foundation. And she did a good job. She didn't know what the outcome was going to be. But she, herself, told me that "Fred, don't worry about the canal." I said, "What do you mean about the canal?" I made a canal that was a serpentine structure. It was like a snake because the yard was very dirty and I put water in it with sticks and branches off of trees. I expected to have trees growing the next day and the water flowing but it didn't happen that way. So she said one day you're going to build a canal that would never dry out. And I have it right here at the village of Usha, 50 years later of that statement. So, my grandmother I know for certain resonated with me, even after she was gone. After she was buried I would still appeal to her wisdom and I would always come up with the answer.

Beverly: What was her foundation? What drove her?

Dr. Sebi: I will never know what drove my grandmother because it was innate in her because her grandmother lived 70 years without a man. Her mother lived 68 years without a man. She lived 65 years without a man and didn't care about it. So I am a product of these four Black women—Violet, Mama Hay, Carolina and Elizabeth, who is my great, great grandmother. I resonate with these women because these women provided a life for themselves without the aid of a man. So, that's why my grandmother told me you don't need anyone and you don't need anything. And if the day comes and you find yourself without clothes you're going to walk as God made you, with the same dignity. So, hey, nothing could happen to me that would make me feel bad because I'm satisfied with nothing. So the foundation of Mama Hay, the only thing I could say is self-assurance, something that you do not find now or very seldom find. Yes, you can. There's a woman that has done things in the United States like Ms. [Mary McLeod] Bethune, like many others in the revolution and the slavery thing, the underground, okay, Harriet Tubman. So there have been women all through history, not only grandparents that I relate to. In fact I would make this clear, I've always resented the voice of a male in my ear telling me to do something. I have never respected the voice of a male dictating to me. I only listen to women, my grandparents. And when they stopped giving it to me I stopped listening. I had what I needed. And evidently it must have been good because I didn't go to school either and here I am curing AIDS. I'm curing sickle cell anemia. How did that happen? It happened out of the cosmic procession, the environment provided for me by grandmother.

Beverly: You said she was powerful but she was never invited to anything.

Dr. Sebi: No, because she didn't allow herself to be invited to anything. She put a barrier around her. She lived that private.

Beverly: Did the shooting have anything to do with that?

Dr. Sebi: The what?

Beverly: The shooting, when she was shot in her breast?

Dr. Sebi: No. When Mama Hay left Belize the man went to jail for life. She wasn't afraid of that. She came here and she was going to the marketplace and do whatever it

10

is she wanted to do and she traveled in Honduras. And she had a business.

Beverly: What was her business?

Dr. Sebi: Seamstress.

Beverly: Seamstress, wow.

Dr. Sebi: Okay.

Beverly: Sara Phillips and her interesting house.

Dr. Sebi: Sara Phillips wanted me to live with her for a while. But I wasn't comfortable with Sara Phillips. Although Sara Phillips lived in a house with rooms and toilets upstairs, and we had to go to outhouses with my grandmother, I wasn't satisfied. I could feel that there was something I didn't like about Sara Phillips.

Beverly: She was on your father's side.

Dr. Sebi: Yeah, my father's mother. Certain things I didn't really learn to digest. It wasn't too palatable.

Beverly: How did you get to her house?

Dr. Sebi: It was just across the street.

Beverly: You did live with her for a while.

Dr. Sebi: For a very short period of time. I think a matter of weeks.

Beverly: A few weeks?

Dr. Sebi: Yeah, I think so, maybe weeks. No years, nothing.

Beverly: She didn't have the effect on you that Mama Hay had.

Dr. Sebi: Oh no, no! Mama Hay had all of the influences. All my influences are Mama Hay because Mama Hay gave me what Sara Phillips didn't have to give. Mama Hay had love. Mama Hay had compassion. Mama Hay was sweet. I could see her smiling with this gap tooth, you know, a big gap in front of her tooth, between her two front teeth. I could see that. I don't remember seeing Sara Phillips smiling. I saw Mama Hay smiling all the time, yeah.

Beverly: Mama Hay, is that her real name?

Dr. Sebi: Her name is Ann Hay. But they call her Mama Hay because she took on that persona only because she used to play these cards. And I used to wonder why this woman play these cards. And I remember these tarot cards. And people used to come with tears in their eyes and they used to leave smiling. My grandmother told me that I should always make them smile Fred. But I didn't know she was using psychology. She knew that the cards didn't have the answers to anybody's problems. She knew that. But what she had to her avail was the sight to see where this person was psychologically. And she would give them exactly what they wanted to hear. Yeah, that's Mama Hay.

Beverly: Fatherhood?

Dr. Sebi: I never had fatherhood. I never had a man to tell me anything in my life. I never heard the voice of a man dictating to me. So, I don't know anything about fatherhood. I just gave my children what was given to me by my parents. Fatherhood? I know nothing about it. I know about grandmotherhood and motherhood; fatherhood nothing. And I suppose that, there, again,

12

nature had it arranged that I was not supposed to hear the voice of a male in my ears. What would I have learned from that male? Males talk to males now. But all the males that talk to males, none of them are doing what I'm doing in other areas, except one—Spaceman! He didn't go to school. But he made an APS, an alternative power source that would last 28 years in your house and in your car. But no, I'm supposed to talk about philosophy, not something pragmatic like that. "No, we don't have no time for making clothes and growing the best food, Sebi. We have to sit around and philosophize." So I only listen to women. No, fatherhood meant nothing to me. I don't know about it. I never had it to say fatherhood. I don't know what fatherhood is. When I look at the natural life expression, I don't see any ducks following drakes. I don't see lion cubs following lion. I don't see gorillas, I don't see elephant cubs following males. So this fatherhood is another American invention that I know nothing about. Nature doesn't show fatherhood. Nature only show motherhood, only. That's why you see, my thinking help me to get this and I did it with ease. "Boy, you're supposed to have some more." And suppose other people had thinking patterns attached to the African resonance. I wonder what they would do? I did it with two women. There again, there again it may sound like I'm putting men down, no. How can I put men down when I'm one? I'd be crazy. But what I'm seeing and what I've always seen, that we males compared to females, we're helpless. You are more equitable and that is shown all through the jungles and even in plants.

Monday, November 7, 2005

Dr. Sebi: In the house that I was raised I always heard that self-preservation was the first law of nature. Being that I am of an African genetical structure, an African heritage, I couldn't very well say Japan or Europe. I had to say Africa, that is the beauty of each and every one of us that represent that gene. That is the beauty. Like the zebra doesn't have babies with horses. They have babies with zebras, alone. And they think of zebras, alone. Orangutans don't have babies with gorillas. No, they do not. So with me saying I'm going to go to Africa, it was an automatic thing. It wasn't something I had to think about. It was automatic because it was ingrained in the house in which I was raised.

Beverly: Your mother or Mama Hay?

Dr. Sebi: Mama Hay.

Beverly: What did she say about Africa?

Dr. Sebi: Well, all she had to say was that we are Africans and she kept saying that. We are Africans. We are not Mayans. We are not Native Americans. We are Africans brought to this part of the world.

Beverly: She told you that?

Dr. Sebi: Um hum. It's as simple as that. I'm an African. I'm not an African-Honduran, no. I'm an African in Honduras.

Beverly: By telling your mother you were going to Africa did you feel like you were going home?

Dr. Sebi: Um hum, exactly. I felt that I was going home. And I felt that. And the first country was South Africa.

Beverly: You have a point you want to make.

Dr. Sebi: The point is that you asked where did substance, the component or what was given by grandmother to me to lay the foundation that I have.

14

Mama Hay—Beginnings

Well, I couldn't give you an answer at the time you asked the question. But as I look back in retrospect, I could remember this: that people would ask my grandmother, "Miss Ann, what's going to happen with Fred?" My grandmother would say, "I don't know." "Miss Ann, what's going to happen to Fred?" "I don't know." "Fred, what is it you want to be?" they would ask me. I said I don't know, because I don't know. I'm only 8 or 9. I didn't know what I wanted to be. "But why don't you go to school, Fred?" "I don't like it." As simple as that. I didn't like it. Okay. What I see now that avails me the privilege to look at things from outside the box, I was never in the box, because I had the freedom to think as I wish for myself. And that is something children are not afforded. That's the one thing Mama Hay afforded me, that environment to think for Fred.

Beverly: I'm glad you mentioned that.

Dr. Sebi: Everybody resonates differently. And everybody comes with a good message afforded in a different way. My grandmother wasn't better than your mother or grandmother either. My grandmother isn't better or worse than any other grandmother. My grandmother just resonated differently. This is what we have failed to see. We always measure things with up and down and good and bad and in between. No. Things are different. How can you compare a lion with a jaguar? They are different animals, to do different things, to live in different geographies. That's another thing about geographies. Plants live in geographies. You would never find a coconut plant growing in Canada. But you'll never find burdock growing in Honduras. So you see, these simple, natural cosmic rules and laws, we don't know about in America. And those laws are the ones that still continue to govern things. So you see, Mama Hay obeyed the laws of life and she transposed that into her grandson. This is why many have asked to change the title of the book but it had to be Mama Hay because Mama Hay was a woman that really had a lot of love and respect for herself. And there is a woman who used to come by and argue with my grandmother. She was the wife of a man who later became the Vice President of Honduras. Her name is Doña Gallarda. Doña Gallarda used to come and argue with Mama Hay about things and politics and racial and all that. But Doña Gallarda always came by and argued and she would come back and argue again and again. And this woman was considered to be one of the elite people of the city of La Ceiba. Doña Gallarda's husband was known as Enrique Ortez Pinel, who was considered to be one of the most intelligent men in Honduras and who later became the vice president to Ramón Villeda Morales. This man's wife used to come and argue with my grandmother and my grandmother used to be telling me about all this and how this woman didn't want to see my grandmother's point and my grandmother couldn't see hers. But I can understand that because they represented two different cultures. That's all. We digest information and process information differently.

Beverly: What did Mama Hay cook? What was the environment like?

Dr. Sebi: The environment in what sense? It was all, the streets were dirt, except now they are paved.

Beverly: The mountains that we see.

Dr. Sebi: The mountains were always there.

Beverly: Very tropical?

Dr. Sebi: They are less tropical now. They are less. There is less moisture in the air than when I was a child. Because right here in the little village of Jutiapa it used

16

to be cold, cold, cold where I had to wear a sweater. And you couldn't see five feet in front of you. The fog was so thick. Now, there's no fog and it's warm because they cut the trees down. But basically, you still have the moisture, the fauna, the flora that one expects to exist in a tropical country, still here. And I guess I enjoy that.

Beverly: What did Mama Hay cook for you? And your mother?

Dr. Sebi: The same thing every grandmother and mother cook today, rice, beans, potatoes, yams, hog feet, hog head, chicken, oxtail. Everything that you see on the table hasn't changed in 500 years. But I was able to get away from it because someone in Mexico said I wasn't honoring my mother or father. And he stopped me from eating meat and because of that I was able to see the other part of it. But she cooked the same thing. That's all she had. And even if she wanted to cook something else, they didn't have spelt in Honduras.

Beverly: Was she alive to see you become Dr. Sebi?

Dr. Sebi: No. She was alive to see me become an engineer.

Beverly: Steam Engineer?

Dr. Sebi: Yeah.

Beverly: When did she pass? What age?

Dr. Sebi: At 100.

Beverly: You were in the states at that time?

Dr. Sebi: Yes. But I got the message.

Beverly: Did you come back for the funeral?

Dr. Sebi: No. I couldn't because when I got the message to make reservations and come to the funeral she would have been buried already, because they only keep you 24 hours.

Beverly: Who are your siblings?

Dr. Sebi: Allen and Felix and then came Maxine, my sister. But Allen was the one after me then Felix. Allen became a mechanic and Felix became a preacher. Maxine, the girl, she got married and then there's John, the last one. The two after me died. The two after them are living. Maxine and John and myself. I'm the eldest.

Beverly: Maxine and John, are they in La Ceiba?

Dr. Sebi: No. Maxine lives in Memphis. John is a businessman. He owns boats that travel the ocean. He's in Venezuela.

~~~~~~~~~~~~~~~~~~~~~~~~~~~~~~~~~~

Young "Fred" Bowman
in La Ceiba

~~~~~~~~~~~~~~~~~~~~~~~~~~~~~~~~~~

Young "Fred" Bowman in La Ceiba

Beverly: You organized the caddies. Tell me about that experience. This is the golf course?

Dr. Sebi: Right there, the same one. The D'Antoni Golf Course. What happened is that there was a little lady here, she was the daughter of Leonard. Her name was Ruth Leonard. Ruth was very sassy. She was the kind of lady that condescends on everyone. So I was a little bit tired of that. So I told the guys, look there's a strike. We going up 100 percent on the tariff. So she asked Chewy who was the leader of this strike. Chewy didn't tell. She said, "Well, I'm going to tell daddy." She went home and told her daddy and he came. That's when Magwa pinpoint me as the culprit that caused the strike. It was good enough that they were paying such a small wage, which was about, in American money, 10 cents a round for 9 holes. Well I didn't feel that her attitude was supposed to be the attitude that she displayed because already we doing her a favor. Because in the tropics we didn't have to carry any golf bag. We didn't need to carry any golf bag because in the tropics you can always find food and shelter. That's one thing. So it was the first time that I hit someone with my hand, when I hit Magwa. I felt he betrayed us all when he pinpoint me.

Beverly: When you say all of us you mean the rest of the caddies?

Dr. Sebi: All the rest of the caddies. But we got what we wanted anyway. But the thing is it showed way back in my youth that there's always the propensity for someone to do something contrary to his own existence.

Beverly: What did you get?

Dr. Sebi: I left because I went to Miramar. I went to work in a dairy farm. I went to work in a dairy farm because I could see there was going to be more confrontation with me and I didn't want that. You see what happened with me, it was never to offend anyone. And I don't have a record of that. I don't know what the result is going to be of that. I can't tell you whether I'm going to chop your head off or whether I'm going to say thanks. I don't know. So I don't put myself in the position of offending someone because I don't know what the response is going to be. So I make sure that I please everyone because I know how I am. I don't know how other people are.

Beverly: Do you play golf now?

Dr. Sebi: I was exposed to golf because I was a caddie. And many, many PGA players were caddies because they got to understand the game, the number of the club with the distance they need to hit that ball.

Beverly: You still play today?

Dr. Sebi: No, well, I stopped that about 25 years ago. I stopped playing golf because I don't have the time. I don't have the time. All my time has been consumed with traveling, building, lecturing. So to play golf, I don't know when that would be. In fact, at this point in my life I don't believe that I would give golf any of my energy because my energy is being utilized with me. Golf is not part of the stuff.

Beverly: Why did you take it up?

Dr. Sebi: I suppose the experience. I played golf for a little while in Los Angeles on Western and Imperial.

Beverly: When you worked at MLK Hospital?

Dr. Sebi: Yeh, when I worked at King Hospital. I used to go play golf with other players. I was never that good. I was never that bad.

Beverly: How often did you play?

Dr. Sebi: I used to play every evening when I worked the swing shift.

Beverly: Really?

Dr. Sebi: Because I'd be off at 2:00. Not the swing shift, the morning shift. I go to work at 6. I'm off at 2. Then I stop at the golf course and I play. I say, leave the golf course at 5:30.

Beverly: So you'd play about 3 hours.

Dr. Sebi: I'd play 9 holes; on weekends I may play 18.

Beverly: What was your score? Your average?

Dr. Sebi: I was no where close to 64. I was more like 74 and 80 or 78 not 80. But that's not even good for an amateur.

Beverly: Not good for an amateur?

Dr. Sebi: No.

Beverly: What's the best score? A Tiger Woods kind of score?

Dr. Sebi: 64, 65.

Beverly: You left caddying and went to work for the Standard Fruit Company.

Dr. Sebi: The dairy farm.

Beverly: The dairy farm was run by the Standard Fruit Company?

Dr. Sebi: Right. It was owned by the Standard Fruit Company. And then I left. I worked there for one year and then I went to work at the commissary.

Beverly: You mentioned two men that supervised you when you were working at the Standard Fruit Company. Why did you mention them?

Dr. Sebi: Montel.

Beverly: and Owens right?

Dr. Sebi: Right.

Beverly: Did they leave an impression on you?

Dr. Sebi: No. That was the first job I ever had.

Beverly: Do you remember their first names? What exactly did you do on the dairy farm?

Dr. Sebi: I had to help with the meat, cutting of the meat, frying of the cracklings. I had to be grinding meat. That's how I lost the tip of this finger—grinding meat, because Aurelio Peralta, he want to elope with this girl. But the girl's mother couldn't stand him around her house. But she could stand me. So he sent me to tell the girl she should prepare herself because he was going to come and get her and run away with her, and that she should throw her clothes, you know, throw her clothes to the window. He was going to come and pick it up. That's how it happened. But while he was talking about it I was grinding this meat. And I stuck my finger in the mill. Oh boy, yeah.

Beverly: That sounds like the movie "Moonstruck." He lost a whole hand. It was funny?

Dr. Sebi: It was funny because you know with us everything is funny. We don't really take things in a serious way. We, hey, it was cool. And then he was married to her all his life and he had all these babies.

~~~~~~~~~~~~~~~~~~~~~~~~~~~~~~~~~~~~~~

United States—New Beginnings

~~~~~~~~~~~~~~~~~~~~~~~~~~~~~~~~~~~~~~

Beverly: So you went to South Africa for the first time in your 20s.

Dr. Sebi: Um hum.

Beverly: Wow. Why South Africa?

Dr. Sebi: I was a merchant seaman. I had to go where the ship goes.

Beverly: You became a merchant seaman because you could travel to Africa?

Dr. Sebi: Because I could travel the world.

Beverly: The world?

Dr. Sebi: Um hum.

I met many people and I learned the value of interacting with different ethnic groups and nationalities. I learned about their customs and food because I traveled to their countries: the Philippine Islands, Arabia, Turkey, India, Russia. I also went to many countries in South America: Brazil, Colombia, Venezuela, Peru, Chile, Argentina, Ecuador, and Panama in Central America. I traveled frequently; first, transporting bananas from Ecuador and later transporting passengers to Brazil and Argentina.

Beverly: By being a merchant seaman you would eventually end up going to Africa.

Dr. Sebi: Most certainly.

Beverly: What does a merchant seaman do?

Dr. Sebi: It does a lot of things. The ship takes cargo. You have people work in the steward department. You have people work in the deck department. You have people work in the engine department. I chose the engine.

Beverly: Engine department? Why?

Dr. Sebi: Because I was always interested in engines.

Beverly: Who instilled that in you?

Dr. Sebi: Nobody. I just had that in me.

Beverly: What was it like to travel to South Africa during apartheid?

Dr. Sebi: I gave a brother a pants and a shirt. This was Port Elizabeth and the police told the brother he couldn't come off the ship with that. So I had to put it on under my clothes to come off the dock to give it to the brother.

Beverly: What did that mean?

Dr. Sebi: It meant that a Black man could not help another Black man. But it's evident now. Right now a Black man cannot go and help any African Black people even though you have the answer to this terrible condition.

It is 1954 and I am taken to the United States on a ship. The city of New Orleans is my first home in the United States, the city where I met Barbara Diggs and lost my virginity. She took me under her wing and helped me ease my way into this new and very foreign culture. She taught me how to talk and dress and helped me understand football. Her family treated me as one of their own.

United States—New Beginnings

Dr. Sebi: Barbara was a beautiful young lady. I was excited. I was excited with her because I never had a girlfriend before. She kissed me. And Barbara used to do that quite frequently and I used to be afraid of Barbara if anything else.

Beverly: Why afraid?

Dr. Sebi: Because I was a country boy from Honduras. She [Matun] met Barbara Diggs's mother. And they're both Aries.

Beverly: Matun, you met Barbara Diggs's mother?

Matun: Yeah.

Dr. Sebi: Ms. Genevieve Diggs, 84 years old wearing hot pants.

Beverly: Oh no.

Matun: Yes she did.

Dr. Sebi: And does she look good?

Matun: She looks real good.

Dr. Sebi: No stuff. Ms. Diggs ain't playing.

Matun: Running behind her grandchildren.

Beverly: How many?

Matun: Her great grandchildren she's running behind.

Dr. Sebi: Ms. Diggs terrible.

Beverly: Really?

Dr. Sebi: Oh look, that's a terrible lady. That's my girl though. I always take her a little salve and Tata tonic. And she likes it. And I love her. I have to love this lady. I feel that way about her. It's like, I remember going to her house and she feeling me.

Beverly: When you first arrived there?

Dr. Sebi: When I was living around the corner from her because I used to live on Pauger.

Beverly: Where?

Dr. Sebi: Pauger Street. P-a-u-g-e-r. I used to live on Pauger. Boy, I remember that too. Right? And that's 51, 52 years ago.

Beverly: You have a good memory.

Dr. Sebi: What you mean a good memory? You cut it out. So Ms. Diggs used to probably know I didn't have anything to eat. I may have looked starved out. And she'd give me some rice and beans and neck bones and some taters. And boy she didn't know how many times I used to leave out of there with a smile on my face. I had me some neck bones and some rice and beans. Yeah.

I was traveling the world and bringing Barbara gifts from exotic places. I was happy and thought she was too, until the day she told me that she was leaving me. She wanted a man in her bed, not one that spent most of his time on a ship. I understood. Barbara is no longer with us, but I will always love her and appreciate her kindness.

Dr. Sebi: She didn't want me on no ships. I came back from my trip—I went to Havana, then Panama, then Ecuador and back. That trip usually took us 21 days.

When I came back she had a boyfriend named Floyd McKissick from Austin, Texas. They fell in love and they had three beautiful children. They have one named Jessica, and the other one named Monica, and the other one name I forgot. But they had these three beautiful childen and I used to visit them. And as I visit them after I left New Orleans I would always go back to New Orleans to visit Floyd. And he loved her. So one trip, hell broke loose with us—them and me or me and them. I had come into the understanding of health.

Beverly: Health?

Dr. Sebi: Yes. And I went back to New Orleans and I caught them eating these neck bones and these chitterlings and this stuff they call, uh, it was pig feet and rice and beans. Pig feet, that's what they were eating. Pig feet. And they were eating neck bones. I said, "Hey, don't do this no more. Floyd, Barbara, don't eat this way anymore."

Beverly: Did she die because...

Dr. Sebi: So Floyd said, Floyd laughed as if I was the loser because he caught up with Barbara. He wind up with Barbara, right?

Beverly: Right.

Dr. Sebi: He thought I was jealous. I said no man. I love Barbara. I said Floyd I will always love Barbara. And my love for Barbara is the same love I have for you Floyd. "What do you mean?" "Stop eating this shit! That's what." And they laughed. Two years later she had a quadruple heart bypass. A year later, she was gone. Barbara passed.

Another thing I remember about New Orleans that was very striking that still remains a memory was a tune. The first American tune that I heard was at a bar known as the Astoria. The Astoria Bar—anyone from New Orleans would verify this—it was on the corner of Gravier and Rampart, North Rampart. There was the Astoria Bar. And in the Astoria Bar I heard this tune, *Casanova*. I don't know if it was Ella, Sara Vaughan or who, but it was one of the most beautifullest tune I ever heard. Oh, I would like to hear it again. It made me feel so good when I used to hear it. I remember buying the White Castle hamburger for 14¢.

Beverly: 14¢? Wow.

Dr. Sebi: Oh yes. We used to buy five. The hamburgers were so small, two bites and they gone.

Beverly: I loved those fried onions.

Dr. Sebi: That's what topped it off. Then we used to go by the Plum Room to eat. This is a plate; it was a little plate: platter with rice and beans and a piece of pork meat in it, with two slices of bread. Now look, the meat is starch. The rice is starch. And the bread is starch. And the piece of meat with a bone in it. So that plate used to cost, I remember how much it cost, 26¢, a quarter and a penny. And we used to go there and buy the root beer with the dinner. Oh wow, beans and rice and meat and two slices of bread and we thought we were batting a thousand, picking our teeth and stuff. So I lived that in New Orleans. I also lived where I had to go on London Canal when I lived on St. Anthony, and get crayfish and buy a pound of rice. I cooked my crayfish and eat my rice and I had a meal.

Beverly: Really?

Dr. Sebi: Tell me I wasn't eating—high on the hog. But New Orleans was beautiful. I loved New Orleans. I love New Orleans now. And every time I go to New Orleans I get the sensation as though I never left.

When I left Honduras and I went to New Orleans it was a quality of love that was being afforded and expressed in New Orleans. This I do not see now. There was a love. There was a closeness and the closeness was because we were being discriminated. It was the most beautifullest thing. When we had to make a decision to go out, we only could go to a Black restaurant. We only could go to a Black theatre. We only could go to a Black anything. But because of that we were closer. I got hooked up with the barbershop, Tim's Barbershop, because I liked the energy there. And these brothers were the ones who introduced me to Islam. They were talking this strong thing that I associated with [Marcus] Garvey.

Beverly: The guys in the barbershop, who owned the barbershop, were Muslim?

Dr. Sebi: Yeah. That's right.

Beverly: They invited you to a meeting?

Dr. Sebi: Finally I went to it. But there was another influence. It was jazz. I met Coltrane. I met Duke Ellington. I met a whole bunch of people because of Tim's Barbershop. He used to do conk, wave hair. I met Roy Hamilton. I met this brother named, what is his name? That used to sing, come on, from Detroit. He used to sing *Summertime*. I used to like to hear him sing that. He was a beautiful singing brother too. Sam Cooke! I would see the Platters and Little Richard. That was the music I listened to when I was in New Orleans because it was just in the 50s. It was on. New Orleans was where I began to grow.

Seven Days in Usha Village

When I was in the Nation of Islam I loved the Nation of Islam then. I love the Nation of Islam now. I will always love the Nation of Islam because what I received in the Nation of Islam I could only have received it in the Nation of Islam. There were components that the Nation of Islam offered that the other entities, religious or philosophical, did not have to offer. But it was offered in the Nation of Islam. At the time that I was a Muslim, it was in the middle 50s. Then, it was a different air about the Brothers. We were happy and the community loved us. The Christian community loved us in New Orleans and we loved the Christian community. We even bought a vegetable truck to bring them fresh vegetables every day. We would pick up their clothes because the Christians were the ones that gave us their business, you understand. So I cannot see why there should not be love among the Christians and the Muslims because as you know, as you and I both know, if I love Muslims and Christians, hey, that's beautiful, it makes it easy for me.

Beverly: So what attracted you to the Nation of Islam?

Dr. Sebi: What attracted me to the Nation of Islam is that I grew up in a Garvey house. And growing up in a Garvey house you get this pride, this sense of value that you add to yourself, that this Black man that you are following could do these great things. So I automatically took on that particular persona because my grandmother was one hell of a Black woman. She was uncompromising. She didn't care how big or how small you were. In her eyes you were the same. But she had this sense of value about herself that I seldom see in people. There are people out there in the United States that have this same feeling about themselves. So when I came to America, coming from this house of Garvey, well, yes, independence is the thing of the day. Sure I was happy when I heard about the messenger Elijah

Muhammad was going to construct schools, farms, hospitals. Well naturally, fresh out of a Garvey house, I am attracted to this, you know like, it's a magnet now, you know, there's affinity, and I love it. I love Malcolm. I love Elijah and I sit at the table at 3837 S. Woodlawn Avenue in Chicago at Messenger Elijah Muhammad house and sat and ate with the holy apostle. And he asked me where I was from. I said I was from Honduras.

"Oh, you came from the land of Garvey. Did you know that Garvey and I are friends? I know him well and that the Mahdi asked Garvey first if he should be the Messenger but Garvey refused," he said.

But you know, we have a tendency to pit Elijah against Garvey, Garvey against Malcolm, King against Noble Drew Ali. No. All of our brothers, all of our brothers and sisters that came to us, came to us with different givings to serve different areas of our struggle, of our journey. I don't call it struggle either because I never use that word struggle. I never struggled in my life, our journey.

I met Brother Malcolm many times and had great respect for him as well as for the Minister Elijah Muhammad. Minister Muhammad was correct in removing the members of the Nation from pork, a filthy animal; but he left the lamb, the beans and all of the starches and sugars. He did the best he could with the information available and his gift is appreciated but I knew it wasn't enough so I left Islam too.

Sunday, November 6, 2005

Dr. Sebi: I remember being in this place and thinking about my life, how I, Sebi—at the time I was Alfredo, not Sebi yet—how I, without knowing, neglected my body and find myself in a mental health institution. But even though I was in an institution being treated, something in me kept saying, you're not going to give up to this.

37

And I wouldn't drink the medication. I would pretend that I was drinking it. And I would throw it away.

Beverly: Why did you agree to being admitted?

Dr. Sebi: It's not that I agreed. I didn't agree to go in. This happened because I was on my way to India on a ship and some reason there was some oil on the deck of the ship and I slipped on it and hurt my spine. And they took me off the ship. But while I was off the ship, the doctor at the hospital detected something in me. His medical report, his final analysis was that I was schizophrenic and paranoid. The man, Dr. King was his name, he was a white man. He was...

Beverly: On the ship?

Dr. Sebi: This happened in the Azores Islands. The ship put me off in the Azores. The ship was on the way to India but I didn't reach India. I am still looking for those monies due to me now. This is 1961 that that happened. They put me off in the Azores Islands and I was diagnosed as schizophrenic and paranoid. When they shipped me back to the United States, I was shipped back handcuffed to a stretcher.

Beverly: Why? What were you doing to make them think you were mentally off based?

Dr. Sebi: I don't know.

Beverly: Were you saying something?

Dr. Sebi: I don't remember that. But as you know, that when you are sick mentally or emotionally you are totally unaware as to your behavior. But I was aware, sufficient to walk out of that hospital. Malcolm was the one who took me out. Malcolm X, the Malcolm that everybody talks about. You see at the time I was a Muslim. So I went to the orderly and I asked him for 10 cents. And he said who are you going to call, your friend, your Martian friends? Oh Bowman has some Martian friends. I say yes, I have some Martian friends.

Beverly: Where did that come from?

Dr. Sebi: Well, he invented that, the orderly. So he gave me the dime and I went to the phone and I called the Mosque. And Captain Joseph answered the phone. He remembered me vaguely but he did remember something of me when I came from New Orleans to Number 7, Mosque Number 7 in New York. He remembered me. So he said he would tell the Minister. And the next day, which was Saturday, I had two baldheaded Muslim lawyers there and they took me out. That's right. They even gave me a state test, the sanity test, and I passed it in front of them. But I knew even though I passed the test that something was occurring in me that needed to be treated. I was aware of that.

Beverly: You knew that something was going on with you. Do you think the doctors were picking up on that?

Dr. Sebi: Right. That's what I said, whatever they picked up for them to conclude that I was mentally helpless or ill, was true, that I didn't know about. I didn't know but I felt it. I don't know what I projected. That I will never know, something, I was very uneasy, I was totally dissatisfied and I used to cry every evening.

Beverly: Your lifestyle? Maybe it's because you weren't doing what you were supposed to do.

Dr. Sebi: If I wasn't supposed to be crying and going through those trials and tribulations I was going through, how was those things occurring?

Seven Days in Usha Village

Beverly: Why do you think they were occurring?

Dr. Sebi: Because they were suppose to occur.

Beverly: They were suppose to?

Dr. Sebi: If they weren't suppose to occur they would not have been occurring. Now the interpretation of the occurrence, that's a different thing. When I never give occurrences interpretations. I just know that whatever occurs in my life was suppose to occur and those occurrences brought me to this end.

Beverly: To where you are today.

Dr. Sebi: To where I am today. Everything was in place when I walked the streets in Baltimore without any money.

Once again Divine Order was revealed when I got a call from a friend of mine in New Orleans about an herbalist in Quina Vaca, Mexico. By this time I knew that nothing was working so I went to see the herbalist. He immediately placed me on an herbal diet along with juice and water for 94 days.

Beverly: And that's what we should do?

Dr. Sebi: We could violate God if we want to. My brother did. If I want to violate God, well, it's up to me. I violate God, but who's going to pay. I'm going to pay. My brother paid with his life but he didn't care.

Beverly: Your brother that was a reverend?

Dr. Sebi: My brother that was a reverend.

Beverly: What was his name?

Dr. Sebi: Felix Gale. Pastor Gale.

Beverly: Felix Gale.

Dr. Sebi: Yeah. And he preached for many, many, many years. Good man here in La Ceiba. That's right at the same place you go last night, the village, the town. But he, my brother, like many other pastors, are not to be blamed for not going to the medicine of the very God they preach about because they were unaware of the devastating impact that glucose would have on the hypothalamus. They were totally unaware. So yes, they love God and they preach God. But they were doing something a little bit different. Because when they get sick, they went to a chemical. That's telling God, God I hear you but I can't do it. And I want everything I said to be written exactly the way I said it. Because that is exactly what's happening. We have to make us aware, hey, look, where are we going with this thing? Look at the rate of murders. Look at the rate of mothers killing their children, one of the things that's unheard of. A mother killing her child? She has to kill. She has to kill her children. Why? She's been compelled to do that.

Beverly: Why do you say compelled?

Dr. Sebi: Because she's eating the things that precipitate that. Yeast will cause you to do diverse things. And I'm going to tell the world this, that at one point there was one of my wives I wanted to kill. Yes, I entertained killing her. Why did I do that and years later I went back to heal her? Because I was healed. The same woman I wanted to kill, I healed her. It is a state of mind.

Beverly: And it's the food we eat?

Dr. Sebi: Well, the food that we eat is the very substance that causes the whole hormonal structure of the body to go haywire because it's of an acid base. So you're going to get acid thoughts. I listened to the guru. I listened to the Dalai Lama. Well, I was not encouraged to any great extent of either one because I know that words do not put you in a cosmic balance. It is the food that you eat that would reconnect you with the energies of life and then words are unnecessary because you could see. You're reconnected. Like the eagle. How come the eagle could make that nest? How come the beaver could make the dam? Not only the spider makes his web. Because it's coded. But you have to be cleansed of the poisons that we were unaware were entering our brain. So now we have to perform. What do you call it, a catharsis? How do you do that? How do you tell someone in Mississippi or even in Honduras or even in Africa around Nigeria, "Say Nigerians, you can't eat gari." Man, he gonna beat you in your head. You cannot tell someone in Louisiana not to eat beans and rice, which is a double negative. You can't tell him that because he's going to hurt you. So, he has chosen death over life. That is what the glucose will do to the hypothalamus.

Beverly: But we don't know.

Dr. Sebi: Well, that makes it even better. You don't know.

Beverly: Why does that make it better?

Dr. Sebi: Because you enjoying your poison. You see, if you knew that you were eating it you'd be chastising yourself every day, because you're unaware. But if you don't know, you're enjoying it. "Yeah man, I like this chop. Man I'm digging this." I remember when I liked my pork chop. I remember when I loved pork chops.

And I remember when I liked eggs, eggs benedict. So when I came into the understanding that these things are dangerous to the body and I would go back to eat them once in a while, I was punished because I know I was doing the wrong thing like before.

Beverly: How were you punished?

Dr. Sebi: I felt bad.

Beverly: Oh, your body reacted.

Dr. Sebi: I felt bad because, no, I felt I'm jive. I'm weak.

Beverly: For eating the poisons again?

Dr. Sebi: That I know are poisons.

After Quina Vaca things began to look better. I felt much better. I was more at ease with myself.

Dr. Sebi: In Mexico, well not to mention Mexico. What I have learned in Mexico there isn't a place in the world that I would give responsibility or credit to for helping me in the area of herbs. There are herbs you find in Mexico that you would never find in the herbal books in the United States, never. They don't even know they exist. But the Mexicans shared those herbs with me and I use those herbs now. I use herbs, that when I talk about them, "I never heard about it." But when you take that position you are taking a position as if you know everything. Well I know as many diseases as we have healed and as many herbs that we have used, we just simply don't know everything. I know my wife and I, we don't want that kind of responsibility. We like having fun and when you know everything, I wonder what that's like. But the Mexican people, the Mexican people showed me something I have never received in any other country in the world, including Africa. They and they alone have the ability to say, when they say how are you doing, when you ask them that, he would always say, "I'm not as good as you. But I'm doing." That's a welcoming feeling, "not as good as you." That's the Mexican. The Mexican, I said, is rooted for certain behavior that long, long ago was taken away from us. We kill our wives. We steal from each other. We have sex with each other's wives. We lie. We, as Matun said, "Who is to be accountable?" You don't have to be accountable to anybody. You do whatever you want. You can betray your race. So what? He made some money. He's rich. Of course he's rich. "The man is rich, man." We sit around and we talk about the black rich people but we never talk about the black healthy people. We never talk about him. The black rich people are more important than black healthy people. Me, I have been in the houses of not only rich people, but presidents and duchesses in France. I'm not impressed. I'm looking for quality of life not positions or richness.

Beverly: How did you get to Martin Luther King Hospital?

Dr. Sebi: A Mexican guy came and told me one day, "So you say you're a steam engineer? Well, if you're a steam engineer how come you're only making $800 a month here, $200 a week? And you're a steam engineer and the county is paying $2,000 plus." I said, "Manuel, where did you get that from?" "Here is the newspaper. And if you're a steam engineer, you're going to teach me how to run this machine." I was operating a corrugated machine at Western Craft in Camarillo. Manuel is the boy name, a young man. He said, "Here it is." I went into the county, passed the test—Building of Safety and something else in downtown LA. Then I went to pass the steam engineer license test. Then they told me there was a job at King and I went there.

United States—New Beginnings

Beverly: You were there for 10 years.

Dr. Sebi: Um hum.

Beverly: What does a steam engineer do?

Dr. Sebi: A steam engineer is an individual that understands the science of thermal dynamics, which is heat exchange. How could you transpose that into healing? Well, yes, because I have to maintain a ph balance of 6.9, which is slightly on the acid side of life. So I concluded that if 6.9 is acid and 7.1 is alkaline, well all the herbs that heal should be on the alkaline side. But when I begin to look at the menus of all the healers in America, they had peppermint, acid. They had aloe vera, acid. They had echinacea, acid. They had dong quai, acid. Every herb that they used, with the exception of a few, like burdock and yellow dock, which are alkaline, and dandelion, the rest of them are acid. So I said well where did Black Americans get their menu from? As I looked at their menu and I looked at the European menu, it is the same. I said oh my God, something is wrong with this picture because they are both in error. But since the black race doesn't have anyone to teach them anything other than the white race, well, naturally they would be subjected to what the white man says is true. But how would they examine what Europe says is true? You don't have any other perspective to put it against to say oh no, this cannot work because I have this as an example. So now you're jammed with that. Well, I didn't have the white man or the Spanish way or the Chinese way. I had nature's way and that's it. So when I was presented with the mechanical way of treating disease I could see the difference because I had the natural way. With the natural way it becomes a barometer. I could measure the unnatural. But if you only have the unnatural, you cannot measure because that's all you have. How would you measure it? You have to have the natural to understand the unnatural. But you don't have the natural. Americans don't have anything about the naturalness of life. So how would they know? How would you know what is natural from what is unnatural? It's not our fault. I'm not saying you willfully deprived yourself of such. The schools didn't have that as part of their curriculum.

I was a steam engineer and I learned from the pH balance of things how to maintain the water. I concluded that if life manifests at 450° F and a pH of 7.1, which is alkaline, then the herbs I said that should heal has to be on the alkaline side of the pH scale. When I look at the Black herbalists in America, from Dr. Llaila Afrika on down to everyone else, they use acid plants. So how come nobody came and pulled their coats? Okay. That's what I'm talking about. But the fact of the matter is because I looked towards Africa, I'm curing AIDS and they are not. You see, because they rejected Mother. When you reject your Mother you reject yourself. And self-abandonment is perpetual blindness. So I want to tell America, Black America, when you reject yourself you are being blinded for the rest of your life. And this is why with the little efforts that I have placed towards Africa, look what we are doing and we're doing it like it was a joke, easy.

I met many friends, on and off my job, but I soon realized that I had to separate from them because our perspective on life, especially food and education, was drastically different.

Beverly: Any Mama Hays in the group?

Dr. Sebi: There was Fumilayo. There was Aduwa. There was Linda and there was another one. And then there were the brothers and the sisters from the other side, on the other side that were professionals: school teachers. And they were like people that graduated from UCLA. I began visiting these two different groups of people as far as purpose in life. What I found was that those that graduated from UCLA and other universities is that they were always deciphering the indecipherable. They were always talking about talking. They used to have these great arguments about this and that about Plato, Aristotle, Diogenes and then they would go into this Black History stuff, never to come out with something pragmatic. The sisters on the other hand, they didn't eat meat. They had these long cotton skirts and when I went to their house, they had these pillows on the floor and they had this incense. And they had these sweet smelling candles. And I was happy because they used to give me these teas that kept me very nice. And I didn't hear any conversation that was in the vacuum of life. Their talk was pragmatic. Their talk is part of what I'm doing now.

Beverly: What did they talk about?

Dr. Sebi: They talked about health, when Black people don't talk about health today. And when they talk about health they talk about it from a Chinese perspective or any other even Indian. But let me remind the world about this, that the Chinese perspective to pathology is offering acid plants such as dong quai. The Japanese that is offering macrobiotic, that's rice. That's cyanide. Then we go to India. The Indian people, with the ayurvedic system of medicine, they tell us to drink cow milk, which is acid. And also rice. So every perspective of medicine that I ever visited and scrutinized, they are all offering us something that instead of helping, they complicate life.

Beverly: You say it doesn't make sense that you're a steam engineer and you're healing people.

Seven Days in Usha Village

Dr. Sebi: When I was a steam engineer at the county of Los Angeles the years were 1970 to 1980. There were healers long before Dr. Sebi doing what they say they were supposed to be doing. All of them, every single last one was doing healing. So how is it that I came last as a steam engineer and AIDS have been cured? And they are not doing that.

When I left MLK in 1980, I was already prepared with the knowledge of compounding herbs and making certain recommendations, which were working to reverse disease. This increased my confidence and enhanced my rapidly growing reputation.

Beverly: Let's talk about the Caribbean. You say you were depressed there.

Dr. Sebi: I was very depressed, not depressed, very depressed, extremely depressed.

Beverly: Dominica was the first place in the Caribbean?

Dr. Sebi: Dominica and then I was kicked out. Then I went to St. Croix. But what I experienced in St. Croix was less than what I expected a brother to afford another brother. Because I live in this dream world where Black people should complement Black people. But that is not the case in St. Croix. In St. Croix the Croixian would let you know "mi bann yah, mi bann yah," letting you know I'm born here. You are not. So you are not welcome. So mi bann yah was told to me many times. And I liked it. I didn't have any problems with it because I know that their experience in life was not my experience in life. You see the people in St. Croix were bought and sold twice by two different countries. So they have two different passports. So that is kind of stressful, to be the property of two different countries and you have no control.

United States—New Beginnings

Beverly: I see.

Dr. Sebi: You understand. So when I went to St. Croix I went into a situation that was not favorable as far as self-acceptance, because of them having that experience of being bought and sold twice.

Beverly: Who were they bought and sold by?

Dr. Sebi: Denmark and United States. Denmark owned it and then they sold it to the United States. So you see, I come from a country that was independent. Do you know when Honduras got its independence? 1824, one hundred and fifty years before any African country. You understand? Honduras been independent ever since then. Haiti been independent since 1821. So coming from the environment that I was raised in, an independent environment, it meant then that I have that independent way about seeing things. I didn't have to go through the stressful situation like the people in St. Croix. I didn't have to pay heed to any government from Denmark. See, I didn't have to do that. I didn't have to pay heed to any government other than the one when I was a child, you understand? It made a lot of difference. So when I went to St. Croix I knew I didn't know the Caribbean Black people. I didn't know that. I was born and raised in Honduras. Their system is totally different, not better, not worse, different.

Beverly: What year did you go there and describe what you saw.

Dr. Sebi: I arrived in St. Croix in 1981 and I stayed until 1983. My first shop was opened up on King Street, on 429 King Street, Frederiksted, St. Croix.

Beverly: Describe the people.

Dr. Sebi: Well, I'm very poor at that. I remember seeing people moving around and about. But because I have never been a judge of people to say "Well, this is what I see and I can judge from what I see this." No. I can't say that about St. Croix. I just saw people. But what I received from St. Croix was, one in particular named Gary. He said that I was a son of a bitch and that I was lying to the people of St. Croix. He said that to me. And other people would throw fecal matter to my window. But all that was okay. I didn't feel bad because I understood that the people of St. Croix were bought and sold by two different countries.

Beverly: Did the fecal matter come before you started healing?

Dr. Sebi: I left Dominica. They kicked me out. Ms. Eugenia Charles, the president of Dominica kicked me out and I went to St. Croix as a place of refuge. And while I was there I received the treatment of fecal matter at my window and telling me to my face I was less than equitable. So I moved to Puerto Rico. And from Puerto Rico I moved to Miami.

Beverly: You experienced frustration the whole two years you were there?

Dr. Sebi: I'm never frustrated. They were frustrated with me. They threw the fecal matter at me. They were the ones that said I was a charlatan, not the US government. The Black people in St. Croix said that. Then it didn't matter to me. It doesn't matter now. Because what I'm going to receive, I'm going to receive and whatever I'm going to receive nobody can prevent me from receiving that. So, St. Croix was two years that I didn't depend on St. Croix. Right? All my business was in Washington and that's when you met me. I didn't do any business with the people of St. Croix. They didn't

50

come to me to buy anything. They would die first. Only one woman, her name is Cleophus Bennett, the only woman in St. Croix and the only being in St. Croix that gave me a word of advice—"Don't be let down."

Beverly: Describe Cleophus.

Dr. Sebi: The Sagittarius woman. The woman that uplift me because definitely I was down because Black people kicked me out of Dominica and Black people disliked me in St. Croix. Ms. Cleophus Bennett was the only woman in St. Croix that came and said I know what you're doing is true. Others may not. But don't let them put you down. And I raised my head for the remaining years and then I left for Puerto Rico, which I was happy to leave St. Croix because how could I live among a people that doesn't exhibit love for themselves? The minute that you dislike a foreigner, you are saying a lot about yourself. Because the one thing that we like in Honduras is to welcome the foreigner.

Beverly: Really?

Dr. Sebi: Are you happy in Honduras? We like that it if you are happy. But in St. Croix, "mi bann yah."

Beverly: So you didn't do any significant healing in St. Croix?

Dr. Sebi: No. Healing who? The Croixians not going to come and see me. Remember I was the Black man that was lying to their parents according to Gary. And he was right. Gary was 100 percent right because that is how he perceived me. I didn't blame the young man. I didn't blame the people that threw the fecal matter at my window. They were right too. You see, everybody's right in my world.

51

Seven Days in Usha Village

Beverly: The crying was because you didn't receive respect from the Croixians?

Dr. Sebi: I wasn't crying because I didn't receive any respect from the Croixians, because I don't need anybody's respect. I don't live by anybody's respect. I don't want anybody's respect. What am I going to do with that? I cannot do anything with that. I was crying because I felt like I was defeated. I was kicked out of Dominica. I was down to $300 and like I failed in the journey, not St. Croix. No.

Beverly: It was the former wife's idea to go to St. Croix?

Dr. Sebi: Yes. She said just go to St. Croix. I said let's go to Miami.

Beverly: Is that so?

Dr. Sebi: Yes.

Beverly: Why did she choose St. Croix?

Dr. Sebi: I don't know.

Beverly: Where is she from?

Dr. Sebi: She's from Africa?

Beverly: She's African?

Dr. Sebi: Yes.

Beverly: What country?

Dr. Sebi: Madagascar.

Beverly: Where the vanilla bean is, right?

Dr. Sebi: The vanilla bean is here too. The vanilla bean is in Grenada more than Madagascar. The vanilla bean is in Nicaragua. The vanilla bean is in Mexico. The vanilla bean is all over. It's a hybrid. It grows all over.

Beverly: I'm familiar with Madagascar.

Dr. Sebi: Madagascar is an island that was chosen to grow spice. But more so in Zanzibar. Zanzibar is the spice island. But Madagascar, you see when we talk about spices, who are the ones that developed these hybrid spices? The French people. Nutmeg, cinnamon, vanilla, all theses things are hybrids.

Beverly: So you left St. Croix and went to Puerto Rico.

Dr. Sebi: Yes.

Beverly: You went to Aruba, Colombia

Dr. Sebi: All that traveling was from St. Croix.

Beverly: You were based in St. Croix.

Dr. Sebi: While doing work in those countries.

Beverly: Washington, DC. How did you get there?

Dr. Sebi: I was invited.

Beverly: I heard it wasn't easy to get you there.

Dr. Sebi: The reason why I didn't want to go to the United States to do any healing, I was doing a very beautiful business between Colombia, Venezuela, Aruba and Curaçao. I was busy with those, and even St. Martin. I had to visit these islands. I was doing well. I was living where it never gets cold. I was living where people you don't have to explain too much for them to understand. Then, I had to leave that and go to the United States. You think I wanted to do that? When I already know that there was going to be heavy opposition against me because I'm Black. So, this young sister said.

Beverly: What was her name?

Dr. Sebi: Adio Kuumba. She said we want you to go to America to Washington and give a speech at the Community Warehouse.

Beverly: Who was she?

Dr. Sebi: Adio Kuumba. I met her in St. Croix. And that's when she heard me saying the things that I was saying and that I could do the things that I said I could do. She went back to Washington and remembered that and invited me to give a speech at the Community Warehouse. And it was a very nice speech. About 700 people came. It was packed and I was happy. But then I got very angry. I got very, very, very angry at the audience in Washington because when I would say things, such as carrots are artificial, they would fight back. I wasn't angry because they fought back. I was angry because they didn't know. I want everybody to know what I know. It doesn't give me any crown on my head to be the one that stands out. The more of us that knows about this, the better life will be for all of us.

Beverly: Why did you come when you were doing so well?

Dr. Sebi: Oh yes.

Beverly: Oh, you're really excited about that.

Dr. Sebi: I was really excited about the Caribbean, doing business in St. Croix, not St. Croix, St. Martin, Aruba, Curaçao, Colombia, Venezuela.   I was happy because those Latin people, they understand medicine. Black America doesn't. Latin America does.

Beverly: You learned healing from them, Mexicans.

Dr. Sebi: Well, I didn't learn it from him. He healed me. I had to put it together.

Beverly: How did Adio convince you to come?

Dr. Sebi: Well, she kept continuing to press me about going to DC and this and that, Black people in America need my service too. And one trip, because I tend to have that same energy as a little boy, I went to DC. I went to New York. The sisters who were living around my surroundings sent me on this mission. When I came back I didn't have any money. They said where's the money? I said the brothers and the sisters said they are going to pay me. Not a person paid me, only one Robert Washington out of New York. And we had to pay rent. And that's when I realized that the women I had around me were really sincere about being around me. They went under the mat and they found 90 cents and they went to the market and they made food that day, with 90 cents.

Beverly: Adio invited you to come right?

Dr. Sebi: Yes.

Beverly: Were you paid for that?

Dr. Sebi: No.

Seven Days in Usha Village

Beverly: Were you supposed to be paid?

Dr. Sebi: No.

Beverly: Did she put up your lodgings?

Dr. Sebi: Yeah, I would stay there. I would stay there but I told them to keep that door. I didn't need the money.

Beverly: Oh, she did collect money from people.

Dr. Sebi: Sometimes they would make up to $7,000 at the door.

Beverly: And you didn't want the money?

Dr. Sebi: No. I didn't want the money. I didn't need it.

Beverly: You spoke free then. It's not like they didn't want to pay you.

Dr. Sebi: They collected. They collected money.

Beverly: They collected money because some of the tickets were like $5, sometimes $10.

Dr. Sebi: That's right. That's correct. They kept that money. I told them to keep it.

Beverly: Okay, it's not like they just didn't pay you.

Dr. Sebi: No. They were very nice to me.

Beverly: What was DC like? '83?

Dr. Sebi: 83.

Beverly: You had never been to DC before?

Dr. Sebi: No.

Beverly: What was your impression of DC in terms of people?

Dr. Sebi: No, but I couldn't expect any response to me. But I loved the people, I love everybody in Washington now, I mean Washington, Chicago and Detroit. They left an everlasting impression on me and Los Angeles, except for you know, where I would say that was not as favorable, Philadelphia. They were very, very responsive. So people all over the United States have been very cooperative with me. And in DC, what I saw was a bunch of beautiful Black people. And I still see that. Jimmy Stroud used to always send people to me and he didn't know me. And after all this time, two years, Jimmy Stroud appears. People used to come and I say who sent you? "Jimmy Stroud." Who sent you? "Jimmy Stroud." Who sent you? "Jimmy Stroud." Then, two years later Jimmy Stroud came and said, "I am Jimmy Stroud." And I love him. He's a beautiful man. Jimmy Stroud is a young man that I would like for all of America to be like, as far as brothers are concerned.

Beverly: And that is?

Dr. Sebi: He's considerate. He's trustworthy. He trusts everyone. He's full of love. He's nothing but love. Jimmy Stroud is a loving person. I felt that of him. He expressed that in his face. You only have to look in his face and you're going to see Jimmy Stroud, all of his soul, right in his face.

Beverly: His daughter, Akili Stroud?

Seven Days in Usha Village

Dr. Sebi: Akili Stroud. He said a lot of people have come and they said some good things about you. You think you can help my daughter? I said I'll try. And we did.

Beverly: What did she have?

Dr. Sebi: She had sickle cell anemia.

Beverly: How did this city run by Black people impress you? Their eating habits?

Dr. Sebi: No, because I lived in countries where Black people run the whole country. So a Black man running DC wasn't impressing to me.

Beverly: What was the response like?

Dr. Sebi: It was favorable. It was good. We always had a packed house.

Beverly: You left Puerto Rico and moved to New York?

Dr. Sebi: No. I had the office in New York but I lived in Puerto Rico. I would board the plane Tuesday morning at 7:00 in San Juan. I would get to New York at 10 and then I would open the place at 11. Saturday evening at 5:00 and 6:00 I closed and get on the plane at 7 to be in Puerto Rico at 10:00 at night and stay home. I would do that every weekend.

Beverly: So when you were lecturing in DC you were living...

Dr. Sebi: in Puerto Rico, yes.

Beverly: So you were commuting between Puerto Rico...

Dr. Sebi: and New York.

Beverly: and even Washington, DC.

Dr. Sebi: Yes.

The Natural and Un-Natural

Beverly: Wheat. Explain how wheat can be manufactured, the carrot.

Dr. Sebi: There again, information. If you are in the position or in the right place to receive that information and then to process that information properly, to process a piece of information requires what? It requires a level of understanding. But like I said to you earlier, that when a child is at a very early age, inception, the first thing that takes place is that they remove the child from his original thinking to that of a school. Once entering the school, yes, he would learn the mechanical way of life. But he would disconnect from the cosmic way of life. And what is the need for the cosmic way of life? It is needed because we are a product of this thing called life procession—the earth. We are a product of such. But when we talk about things like wheat and carrots and beets and turnips, the individual that is able to assimilate that information is an individual who would have had a connection with things outside of the box. In the box wheat is natural. Outside the box wheat is unnatural. Why? Because it contains starch. Nothing in Nature contains starch. And everything that was made by man has to contain starch as a binder. But starch is carbonic acid.

Beverly: Wheat is carbonic acid?

Dr. Sebi: Definitely. Any grain that is made, corn, wheat, rice, these things are starch. Starch is not a food.

59

Starch is a chemical. Starch is what you use to separate region. I did because I'm an engineer. I understand how to use starch. Starch is not a food.

Beverly: So it's manufactured, those wheat, rice and carrots.

Dr. Sebi: They are manufactured. They are manufactured and how are they manufactured? The other part of the story is this, very few people understand that a mule is an artificial animal. Well, naturally, it would be difficult for someone who has been to school to understand such things, that a mule was made by man. Oh come Dr. Sebi, how can man make animals, only God can do that. Well, what man did was to take two of God's products and manipulate them in a way that then he can produce a third product. What do I mean by a third product? Okay. If you take a horse and you take a jackass, you would definitely make a mule. But God didn't make mules. God did not make any mules. Man did. Man made mules. If God wanted mules to be here, God would have made mules but he didn't.

Beverly: What about the cow?

Dr. Sebi: And in nature...

Beverly: Okay.

Dr. Sebi: ...he takes, like in a vegetable, he took the wild yam and the queen anne lace and cross-pollinate them. He opened a sliver of the plant, which is in the stem. He opens a sliver and in there he placed some of the pollen of another plant, which is the queen anne lace and the end product is a carrot. But then he had to rape the wild yam. For you to produce an unnatural product you have to do raping. Raping means

60

Beverly: What do you mean rape?

Dr. Sebi: Rape, because generally plants would not pollinate one but of its own kind. And for you to make a third product that was not made by nature, you have to force this other plant to produce a product that it was not designed to do.

Beverly: Is a carrot a starch though?

Dr. Sebi: A carrot has nothing but starch. If you grate carrot and you grind it, just grind the juice and let it sit, and look what happened at the bottom of the carrot, nothing but starch. It's thick.

Beverly: Okay.

Dr. Sebi: I gave a talk on WLIB in New York at 1:00 with Gary Byrd. And I remember making the statement in New York that a carrot was artificial and everybody in New York thought that I was talking out of my head, that I was out of my mind. And I had to agree with them because the information that they had was limited. Not that my information was so expansive either, but it is a little bit different, coming from a different place. Like I was born in Central America. I grew up in Central America so I could compare the life of the forest and that of a city. But if you're born in a city, all you know is the city. And if you're born in a forest and grew up in a forest, that's all you know. And it's not your fault. But I was born in the forest and experienced the city for some fifty-some odd years. The components of nature that I have experienced, and that of the young man who grew up in Harlem all of his life, those components are unheard of. But likewise, he would tell me things about a city that I know nothing about.

Beverly: Like the cow, you say is not a real animal either.

Dr. Sebi: When we talk about not eating meat, we also have to be very careful. Because in nature we find there are groups who eat meat and there are groups that doesn't. Among the meat eaters you find them on all levels of expression.

Beverly: You mean people?

Dr. Sebi: Every living species.

Beverly: Even animals.

Dr. Sebi: Even animals. You find some that are carnivorous and some that are herbivorous. So just go to the birds, the most delicate of them all. What do they eat? They eat seeds. They eat fruit.

Beverly: Like sparrows.

Dr. Sebi: That's right. But the eagle and the hawk, they eat meat and blood like the bat. He sucks blood. His diet is straight blood. He was made to digest blood, so was the eagle and so was the hawk. But not the hummingbird, not the sparrow. They have nothing to do with that. Now we go to the animals, the gorilla. Man, you don't go putting blood in front of a gorilla. He runs. That's why you don't have to be afraid of a gorilla, because he represents that which he eats. A gorilla? Man, he's cool. The gorilla, he have nothing to do with blood. He eats leaves and berries because his cellular arrangement does not even permit him to think mentally to eat blood. He is coded by nature to eat leaves and berries, not bananas. Ah, not so for the polar bear. This dude, he likes blood. He tears his thing apart. He's just vicious with his stuff. Hey man, you bring me some—the bear of fruits and berries would be consumed by me because I eat meat. I eat blood. That's the polar bear. But the blood that he eats suffice him because he was made to do that. As we leave the bear and the gorilla we go to plants. Plants? Eat meat? Well what about the venus flytrap? Oh-h-h, so even among the vegetarian life you find some that eat meat. Others don't.

Beverly: Because they were encoded to do so.

Dr. Sebi: That's right. But as we leave the vegetarian world, no, as we continue and we leave the plants and the animals and birds, we now direct our attention to the Homo sapiens. Every Homo sapien on the planet eats meat. Something is drastically wrong with that picture. You do not find that in the bird family nor in the animal nor in the plants. How and why do we find this expression among the Homo sapiens, that everybody eats meat? No, not so. What occurs is that we have been taken into a world of philosophy, a world that wants to shape everyone around that one pattern, when that is not seen at any time in nature. You find different colors of expression that needs different food. You find that the blue vervain, the blue vervain is a plant that digests potassium phosphate. And she grows right here in the village and she's a pretty plant. If you want your nerves to be treated properly just think about the blue vervain, the root and the flower. But if you want your bones strong, you have to go to the sea moss, and it will strengthen your calcium cells.

Beverly: When I look at you talking about the plants, you look mesmerized, you look like you're on a high just talking about the plants.

Dr. Sebi: Well, I have to say this, that I think I told you earlier that I didn't want to be a healer because I consider myself vulgar. I consider myself loose, undisciplined, all of those things I feel of myself. And I suppose I feel that way because my measures are my own. That's all I have. I cannot use the yardstick of another because I am unique, like everyone else is unique. So naturally as I look at this arrangement of life I find myself being very extremely careful, careful because I have not ever or do I remember wanting to be anything in my life. I want to be me. In the me, in the wanting to be me, I find that a whole lot of things came out of that, such as the healer. I'm not even convinced that the people who were cured of AIDS have been cured because there was not effort for me doing that. I could see myself doing it. I wonder why others are not doing so. Instead of them sharing with me, which is their responsibility to the world, not to me, because if I afford myself to the world as a healer, and I am not as responsive or I am not affording what others are affording, then it is my duty to visit those that are doing things on a higher level than I to learn how to help in complementing people in need.

Agua Caliente—Usha Village

Dr. Sebi: Curing AIDS? That's the smallest part of what Africa has afforded Sebi. Curing AIDS is the easiest thing.

Beverly: Thermal waters.

Dr. Sebi: The reason why the thermal water is so effective, and it's a very good question, very good question because everybody who comes here they're amazed. They come here with Kaposi's sarcoma. That's the last stage of AIDS, when the sores are on your skin, breaking down your first defense, your skin. They go into the thermal baths and in four days the sores have disappeared as if they were never there. A man came from Argentina with lung cancer, but instead of him going in the bath water, I put him in the sauna where he is now going to inhale the waters and vapors into his lungs. In two months his lung cancer disappeared completely. So now why, why does it have such a calming effect on the body when you lay in it and you go ah-h-h, this is so delicious? It goes to the pores, the high concentration of sulfur, phosphorous and iron. Sulfur is the main ingredient in thermal waters. Sulfur. And sulfur, natural sulfur, because there is a such thing as artificial sulfur. That's the one you give those cows in the barns. Natural sulfur, organic sulfur is the greatest thing for your lungs. The cells of the lungs are made of sulfur. Like the bones are made of calcium. The blood is iron. Sulfur begins to do repairs in the lungs. Phosphorous is the great company for iron, which is going to electrify you and at the same time a calming effect. The pH of thermal waters is 8, 9.6, 8.9, which is extremely high. Any substance that has such a high concentration of hydrogen, iron concentration, hey, it is effective in healing because it is oxygen that heals; nothing else but oxygen. That's why.

Beverly: You say you were really excited about curing AIDS in the 80s. Address that.

Dr. Sebi: Yes, of course. I was happy to know that the perspective that I was using was affording me the privilege to reach that level of offering. I was happy because in the past I had visited Dr. Woo, a Chinese. He didn't heal me. I went to some black herbalists in California. They didn't heal me. And then I went to the chiropractor and he didn't heal me. So naturally when I put it together and I trusted my judgment . . .

Beverly: Put it together? The compounds?

Dr. Sebi: Put the compounds together. I trusted my judgment. Why? Because I selected plants whose molecular structure is complete, which deems them electrical; and so is the human body. But when the individual that had AIDS was cured, Mr. White, then I was encouraged to know or when the blind man was seeing I was further encouraged. So you see, I had to be excited. But the excitement is giving way to reality.

Beverly: And that reality is?

Dr. Sebi: That what I wanted is one thing and what is forthcoming from my brothers and sisters is another. It's totally different. I am not talking about those of us who are sick because the people have come in large quantities, sure. They have been supporting me for the last 30 plus odd years. Sure, and I give all of you thanks, of course. But we are talking about the people who have taken responsibility to lead others. Those were the people. Those are the people that represent the reality that I'm talking about. The reality is yes, Dr. Sebi can cure AIDS and lupus and herpes. But yes, on the other hand, it doesn't mean anything because we're not going to support him. I accept.

Beverly: How are you not supported?

Dr. Sebi: I don't believe that it's necessary to mention names. I'm talking about every Black American leader. That's who I'm talking about. Because they claim that they are leaders. So naturally one expects for a leader to help the flock out of the disease state to a better state. They, not I, took the position of leadership. So if you're going to lead a people, and from the people came the solution to one of the major problems that beset the community, and you do not act on it, what is the message that you are sending? That is the reality of the thing.

You see, I'm not the person you urinate on the head and tell him it's rain. I smell urine. That's why I act the way I act and that's why I have retreated to this because in my not affording myself the way people think I should, well, that's their opinion. I feel joy and happiness right here. I don't even go out of my door sometimes for a month. I do not go out that door. I bathe. Chipita brings my sea moss. I sit here. I look at TV. I look at the patients come and go but I'm not going out that door. So you see, my grandmother and my mother showed me to be satisfied with nothing instead of having to have a lot and still dissatisfied. I'm satisfied with nothing. But my brothers and sisters, this is important because I have been in America for 52 years and I could rightfully say this, that everything that was brought to us in America in the last 52 years were words, a bunch of words. And those who bring words continue to say that words are necessary. Well, if words are necessary there isn't a people on this planet that has had many words beginning with Noble Drew Ali, Father Divine, Daddy Grace, Bishop Jones, Elijah Muhammad, Malcolm X, Martin Luther King, Reverend Butts and many, many, many, many others. Words? I mean, I don't know anybody on this planet that has so many leaders like Black America. And boy they are proficient in words. Oh that I know. They can talk. But when it comes to executing, executing where something is pragmatic—animals don't live philosophy. They only live by the laws of life, doing the things that support their life. But my leaders, no, not my leaders, but the leaders of America, they take you into everything else but life. So therefore we are left hanging because they didn't have that to offer. But I'm saying this, that the glucose we talked about earlier has taken a toll to the extent that I cannot look into the eyes of my sister or brother and see beauty. No. I am suspicious when I look in your eyes because I don't know who you are. And who is this nigga anyway? I have heard this thing a thousand times. And I will repeat it the way it was said, "Who are you nigga? I don't know you." This happened to me in Santa Monica. He slammed the door in my face. The man was right. The man was responding to the dictates of glucose on his brain. There has never been an educator in America that has done research in neuropathology associating the disease with the food that goes in the person's mouth. That research has never been done. But yet I know for a fact that this book is going to raise many eyebrows. Well, let it raise them because they haven't done anything anyway. So what rule do they have to challenge? You see, nobody could challenge me on this planet because I have accomplished what no one else has accomplished. So where's the room for challenge? Since there is no challenge there is ridicule. But I say this, that the glucose on the brain is shown when all of the leaders of America that know about the entities of healing and have turned their backs on it. I can openly say they all know that I exist. I have proof of that too. When I was taken to the Harlem State building [Adam Clayton Powell, Jr. State Office Building] to address AIDS, the African American War on AIDS in 1989, well, I made the stupid move again. I went to the Harlem Building and I told them that I had the cure for AIDS and they laughed. I went to Detroit and I told Dr.

70

Whitner I had the cure for sickle cell anemia. He laughed. I went to some of the biggest leaders in America and they laughed. So now Dr. Sebi knows that healing someone with diseases is one thing, but changing their thought pattern, well. I said that with the removal of the food, like Elijah Muhammad said to us, that they gave us the wrong food to eat. So if there's any change, well, hope there'll be. But changes cannot be accomplished and will not be forthcoming if the diet has not changed. And if the diet is not changed I will live long enough to see that in the next 30 years, America is not going to change.

Sunday, November 6, 2005

Dr. Sebi: The Black man was never supposed to eat meat. And I am going to make this statement, unlike previous people that was made to be afraid of making a statement that is consistent and truthful. The Black race cannot assimilate meat nor alcohol. Why? Because over the 31 years of my research, when my genetic group that I represent, the so-called Black man, the African, I find that when they come with diabetes, lupus, herpes, and this is all manifested in one body, in less than a fortnight, all of the diseases disappear. But we have to abstain from eating the very substance that made our body sick, which is the blood of the animal. Meat was never supposed to be consumed by the Black race. But maybe other races, like I was told in Atlanta. I was told in Atlanta by a Native American at the lecture that I gave recently in the month of October, October 9; this Native American said Dr. Sebi did you know that they found a very rare enzyme in the blood of the buffalo and that enzyme prevents the individual from getting cancer and this is why the Native American people have a very low rate of cancer incidence. So there is a rare enzyme in the blood of the buffalo. I said that may be true for Native Americans but I represent a different gene group and in that difference a lot will be seen and could happen. What occurs is that the difference has never been treated. Over the last 500 years, the intent is to group all of us in obedience to a philosophy. But that does not hold true for the plants, and the flowers and the planet. Even the birds, they all obey the dictate that was designed to support their life and their cellular group. Like it is mentioned, the gorilla does not eat meat. Where did the gorilla get that message from? He didn't go to school to learn from some nutritionist that his cells are not made to digest meat. It is encoded in the gorilla, like everything else. But when we talk about encoded, what is it that we are talking about? We are talking about an expression or an electrical connection with life. That electrical connection is what brings the message that gives you the ability to make a decision that is equitable and good. But when we disconnect from that electrical connection we make mistakes. We are vulnerable. The gorilla never makes mistakes. But human beings, they make mistakes. Because it is seen that the Homo sapien puts meat and cheese in his mouth and I'm referring to those who represent the gene of Africa. But by the time they get to 45 the doctor politely tells them, "Well Mr. Johnson, I find that you are suffering with hypertension. Your pressure is a little high and by the way, did you know that your PSA is a little high?" The Black man, Mr. Johnson, is totally unaware that he's obeying a dictate that had nothing to do with the history of his cellular predisposition. The gorilla didn't go to school. Mr. Johnson did. Mr. Johnson has a master's degree but he didn't know what to put in his mouth. The gorilla, without the degree, because he's still tied to the cosmic procession, then, without the degree, he knows what to eat. This is what I'm talking about. I, Dr. Sebi, am one because I still wear clothes. And I know that that is very offensive. That is where life begins to deteriorate, wearing clothes.

Agua Caliente—Usha Village

Beverly: Wearing clothes?!!

Dr. Sebi: That's right! God did not make clothes. Clothes prevent the cells below your clothes from receiving oxygen. The oxygen that is supposed to be received is deprived because you have clothes on. But the visitors, the visitors, when they came to visit us, they said we were naked. Uh oh, where do you get that word from Mr. Visitor? Because we live like this all our lives. Why do you say we are naked? But in a state of nakedness the violation to a woman does not exist. Everybody was in sync. Everybody was living beautiful. How many of us would like to visit that zone again? Well, let me say this. Recently there is an anthropologist, a white Caucasian Jewish lady that made a statement that she's in search of the super human. So she was asked who is the super human? Who was the super human? Who are these people? She said well, the super human is an individual who doesn't go to the supermarket to buy food. He's insect repellent. He doesn't go to the doctor to get any injection because he only eats vegetables. And the super human is very humble and he doesn't wear any clothes. When she said that I said now isn't this something, that in the year of 1490 or the year of 1300 my ancestors were described as savage. In the year 2005 I am hearing the anthropologist say that they were super humans. So we need to reexamine or revisit the position of our mothers and our fathers. It is said honor thy mother and thy father that thy days may be long upon the land. Well that statement doesn't hold true for a gorilla or an elephant. That statement is totally unnecessary because they follow their mother and their father from the day that they are born, the day that she delivered them. That elephant watch what mother eat and so does the gorilla. Now, with the Homo sapien, the Black race especially, I'm talking for the Black race, the one that they call the African, my gene, we were disconnected from our mothers and our fathers. We don't even know the food that they ate in the jungles of Africa, as they call our place, our dwellings, the jungle. So when the FDA [Food and Drug Administration] wanted to prevent me from products, I politely asked the FDA well, maybe the FDA knows the food that is consistent with my cellular predisposition. When you removed the African from Africa did you bring his food with him? Uh oh, that went by. But what people aren't aware of is that those who deprived us of our food, they once in a while find us behaving a little bit other than what they would like. And for ourselves, we deprive ourselves of those things that would place us in a comfortable place, whether we had money or not. Because we came from a people that didn't have any money. We could live life without money. We could design societies. All it takes is some mud and some grass and we could build empires again. Because we did it right here in the Usha Village. All these huts are mud. They're mud and grass. And we could do it again as easy as that. But being disconnected without knowing the food of our mothers, so that we could live long upon the land, we eat things that offend our bodies. But even that is in place. You know, like Job. He had to get sick before he turned to God. You see everything is in Divine Order. So the European that brought us here was in Divine Order too. But what he didn't know, he brought us here to do a job. He didn't even know the job we were going to do. Our job is to heal them. That's right. Just like in the human body, the cells of the brain are made up of copper and carbon. They do not resemble the cells that make up the bones. They are calcium, not to mention the cells that make up the blood. They are iron. They are different cells and they do different things. So the Black race, the Chinese race, the White race, the Eskimo, the Native American, we all were placed here to perform certain duties. But since there was an interruption in our duties that we were supposed to perform, things seem to get out of hand. As we notice

74

carefully, there's unrest all over. So it is necessary for healing. So the healing is coming from us. Yes, we are proud to be the servant of the world, the Black race. The angry ones turned out to be the cornerstone that the builders needed to complete the structure. And that's true. You see, we denied ourselves because we were given the wrong foods to eat.

This is why Mudsimi Wakanaka has launched or campaigning or trying to develop, say campaigning in the area of providing an environment where people would learn to cook the new food. People learn how to prepare and learn what to select. Industry would just shift but it would still be provided, you understand? They are not going to lose any money because if you don't eat meat, you eat mushrooms. Then industry would begin to grow mushrooms. It's cleaner and it doesn't bring the bovine spreading all over the place. It's cleaner and it's healthier for everyone in question. The providers of the mushroom would make more money and they have a cleaner environment. But right now, their product is poisoning the world. You hear mad cow disease. You're not going to hear mad mushroom disease.

Beverly: So Mudsimi Wakanaka is that arm to teach us how to replace the poisons?

Dr. Sebi: And how to live within the boundaries that would allow peace and tranquillity because it is peace that you're looking for. It isn't money. You could have all the money in the world and if you do not have peace, then acquiring money is of no avail. But if there's peace, man, money could come later. You know, I'm chillin'.

Beverly: Sleep well.

Dr. Sebi: What you mean? I'm chillin'. I'm chillin', okay? But to chill you can't eat a hot dog and say I'm chilling because I know what that hot dog is going to do.

The uric acid is going to play havoc on our what? The central nervous system. But our children are saying, man I'm chillin' but look. It's like the guru and the Dalai Lama. They be telling us about peace, about what we need to do about peace, how to obtain peace. They tell us, right? But when you go home to eat, the very thing you put in your mouth undermines the goal you're pursuing. So that's why I was never impressed with either one.

Beverly: What is that thing that drives us?

Dr. Sebi: When I talk to Spaceman about his invention, the APS, the alternative power source, I never ask Spaceman what was in him to do that. Know why? Because he doesn't know. Spaceman would never know that. All Spaceman knows is he could do it. I said to you one day curing AIDS and lupus and herpes, blindness and diabetes, that is as easy as ABC for me. Now you want me to tell you what prepared me to do this. Oh yeah, I'm a magician now. How would I ever know that when I'm in obedience with that energy? I don't know what it is. I'm in obedience to whatever that is. And I don't question it. I never question me. I remember in my dreams I dream that I fly every day. At night I fly. And when I come back on the ground, oh boy what a relief it is, when I fly. And my life reflects that flying. Because I see things from the top and it becomes easy. Many people are in the forest. They cannot see. I see things from the top. It becomes easy. But when I talk about from the top that becomes confusing now to everyone. By the top I mean that I see things from the top where I can grasp the whole spectrum. I have a larger platform. And I always did that. Like for instance the African people, the African people lived for millions of years without the aid of money. Now the African people find themselves needing money to feed themselves. The African needs to starve to death. All of them need to starve to death. That in itself is telling them that they have departed so far from their ancestors that now they need money, something that was never part of the repertoire of Africa—money. You can't even eat if you don't have money. Well you should starve to death. With me, it would not be that if I was the president of an African country. I would show them but with my understanding of this point now. I'm not saying that the president of Africa knows what I know. They were interested in civics and politics. Mine was a different giving. It was healing as an individual, not as a leader president, as an individual citizen in a country, America or Africa or Honduras. I am indebted to America just as much as Africa or Honduras. I would make certain suggestions. Since we find that the African people are starving because the corn suffered a drought or the wheat, well, that's okay. Let us understand, was the corn really nourishing our body? The answer is no. It was stimulating our body, not nourishing. So now we're going to change this, this format. The paradigm has shifted right? The method has to change. Am I right? So now that Africa finds itself at a deficit financially, well, just go back to the ways of our fathers. Let's go back to the forest and find the herbs that have the energy. And in the meantime we can begin to grow the cotton that makes our clothes. We can begin to experiment with new organically electric food where nobody buys food. No. What you mean you buy food? That's a European thing. That's not an African thing. So Africa live in Europe now. So Africa have to die. Oh I wouldn't mind seeing them die. To you that sounds like a deficit on my part. I'm losing points. No, I'm not losing points. I'm telling you what needs to be. And it's happening now greater than what I expected. They dying by the thousands a day. Okay?!! So they need to die. If they didn't need to die they wouldn't be dying. I wouldn't like to see it but they need to die because we have forsaken our fathers and our mothers. There's no way around it.

And that applies to me. The little that I was able to get out of my mother and my father, it has had me at 72 years of age with a healthy body. Sure I feel good. But I can't transpose that to Africans. They going to die of starvation instead of listening to me. It happened in Zimbabwe. It happened in South Africa. It happened with many places in Africa, including Nigeria. They eating stimulants. They are not nourishing their body.

Beverly: A woman's meal of turkey, gravy, rice, she's asthmatic. How would you treat this lady?

Dr. Sebi: The first thing I would do is what I do for everyone else. To fully understand what we are doing here at Usha Research Institute, we have to understand, again, life's arrangement. Understanding life's arrangement makes it easier and facilitates reversing a disease. Like for instance, I said all that to say this, understanding. We, over 31 years of affording ourselves, we do not treat the disease like the physician or like the nutritionist. We treat the disease biochemically. We know that when disease is present there's a chemical imbalance. Whether there is diabetes, leukemia or sickle cell, cancer, asthma, whatever the disease, we make the same compounds.

Beverly: What are they?

Dr. Sebi: But we have to understand what it is we are going to remove from the body to make the individual recover as quick as possible. In the case of asthmatic, an asthmatic person, the bronchial tubes are clogged. His nasal passage suffers with what? Pneumonia. Quite often he suffers with bronchitis because asthma says that the body has reached a level of mucus accumulation that is insupportable. I should know. I was born with asthma. I was born with asthma and I had asthma until I was 30. But what I learned about asthmatic people,

78

they are neurotic. This is why I found myself in that mental institution, because an asthmatic person, the one thing he is lacking is oxygen. Being deprived of oxygen, he fights to stay alive and then any little thing triggers a reaction that is negative. He cannot have that because the oxygen that keeps one healthy and also stable or tranquil, he's being deprived of it. Not only does he wheeze, he's deprived of the bread of life and a lot occurs when that happens. So an asthmatic person, I'm surprised you asked me about an asthmatic person, people or the disease of asthma because I was saying that when you describe an asthmatic person's condition, you describe all others because all diseases stem from the accumulation of mucus, whether it's in the bronchial tubes that give you asthma or on the brain that makes you insane. In the prostate glands, prostate. And if the same mucus goes to the pancreas, it's diabetes. So yes, we were able to reduce disease to its least common denominator.

Beverly: A change in diet and?

Dr. Sebi: That's most necessary and drinking the compounds.

Beverly: Compounds?

Dr. Sebi: The same thing. Why is that? Because what causes prostate cancer? Inflammation. What is inflammation? The accumulation of mucus.

Beverly: What are the compounds?

Dr. Sebi: The compounds are phosphates. They are carbonates. They are iodides and they are bromides. What do I mean? They fall into the categories of food and vitalizers. And I'm quoting Shook, Edward Shook. He breaks down the minerals better than anyone I ever read or heard of. But where I differ with Shook is that many times Shook used inorganics to accomplish his goals and he used certain herbs that are unnatural, such as he recommends garlic. And garlic is acid. And maybe when he recommended garlic he was recommending for his own gene group.

Beverly: How can a person who doesn't know about herbs and natural foods become aware of this so that he can eat properly? How can he tell a hybrid from a natural plant?

Dr. Sebi: For someone to be prepared or educated to understand that which is natural from that which is unnatural, if we have to do that, boy, it's going to take a million years, 40 million people plus. But how do you afford them? Well, the book is going to spread I suppose and people may get something out of it to apply to their life that would improve the quality of their life because that is all living is about, the quality of your life. How do you educate that person to understand that? I don't know. I simply don't know.

Beverly: What can you teach us now?

Dr. Sebi: I'm going to start with this young lady that came to us. Her feet were going to be severed from her body. Her name is Paula in San Diego. This lady listened to what we had to say. But when you begin to touch upon that, that subject such as changing people's diet so that they can live better and how to help them, you're going to find yourself being the enemy of everyone. But I'm going to take the chance anyway because you want to know. Well, Sister Paula was at an extreme pathological condition. She was septic.

Beverly: Which is?

Dr. Sebi: Her body was riddled with fecal matter and debris, acid, which all of us are. It was manifesting in her feet. But the majority manifests in their skull. She was lucky that it was in her feet, where the acid concentrated. But 99 percent of Black America, it concentrates on their brain. I'm going to prove that. So now how do we help that? Paula came and said I'm dying. They want to cut my legs off because I'm septic, gangrene and the whole bit, poor circulation. I said what's your religion. She said I'm a Muslim. I said are you ready for this? You can't eat bean pies. "Why?" Because the bean pie has eggs. It has sugar, glucose. It has butter, concentrated fat. It has carbonic acid, which is the flour. So now when you put all that together, you have a lethal bomb. But the sister doesn't know it. But the sister is wise. The sister stopped eating the bean pies and the carrots and the rice and beans. She has her feet and she no longer has diabetes. Now when she called, I don't know who she called in the officials in the Islamic world. She said she called Mr. [Louis] Farrakhan. And he just rejected everything that she had to say. So when you ask me the question how do we begin to educate people about their diet, that's an individual thing because what you're going to find is that the good you're trying to do, our leaders will have you hung. So besides the leaders having you hung you have to deal with the deficiency in the brain, which is not going to permit them to change. Like the African people, when you tell an African from Nigeria do not, under any circumstances, put gari in your mouth or cassava, he may slap your face. Yet he's going home to put cyanide on his brain. So how do you do it? I don't know. I am telling my brothers and sisters in America and around the world and for that matter every other race, watch what you eat. Avoid the starch, which is carbonic acid, the uric acid, the lactic acid and there's many more. But avoid them and begin to relax yourself, which I have never heard anyone make this recommendation before.

Beverly: What are some good alkaline foods?

Dr. Sebi: Mushrooms. Then you have spelt. You have quinoa. Those are the grains. Quinoa, teff, the other one from the desert of Mali, which is fonio. And then you have the amaranth. These are natural grains, alkaline.

Beverly: What other foods? These are grains. What vegetables?

Dr. Sebi: Natural spinach that we have growing here at the Village, that you could also have in the United States. I have a natural spinach that runs on a vine that produces a flower.

Beverly: What about collard greens?

Dr. Sebi: No.

Beverly: What?!!

Dr. Sebi: That's very hard on your digestive system.

Beverly: Collard greens?!!

Dr. Sebi: Most definitely.

Beverly: Kale? Mustard greens?

Dr. Sebi: Mustard greens are more digestible. So is kale. Turnip greens too but not collards. They are very hard, very hard.

Beverly: Spinach.

Dr. Sebi: Spinach has a lot of oxalate acid.

Beverly: That's not good?

Dr. Sebi: Well, it's questionable.

Beverly: The starchy foods of course are peanuts and what else?

Dr. Sebi: They have carbonic acid.

Beverly: Tell us a story about starch like your planet cop story.

Dr. Sebi: We shouldn't even single out one or two of the items that you mentioned. Anything that has an acid base will undermine your immune system immediately, primarily because it's an acid base. It's going to eat you up. It's going to weaken the system. It's going to weaken the red blood cells. Acid causes the central nervous system to contract, which again causes you to go into a state of despair. So what are acids? Well, you just walk into a supermarket and walk out with a coconut. Everything you left behind is acid. But there are health food stores that have mushrooms, the portobello. You also have the oyster mushrooms. You also have the spelt bread. You have quinoa. You have amaranth.

Beverly: You went to jail because of your love of plants. Where were you jailed?

Dr. Sebi: St. Martin, Curaçao.

Beverly: Mexico?

Dr. Sebi: ... I was kicked out. Mexico, I went to jail too and then the United States.

Seven Days in Usha Village

Beverly: What happened?

Dr. Sebi: What happened?

Beverly: Yeah. Rarely do you find someone going to jail over plants.

Dr. Sebi: Everything I do is rare. That's why it is comfortable with me. Everything I do is so strange, strange to everyone but me. It's so easy for me. Everything is easy. I didn't put any effort into anything.

Beverly: What happened in St. Martin?

Dr. Sebi: Well, the French didn't want me disseminating my product in their country because St. Martin is divided into two different countries, Dutch, which is Williamstad, French, Marigot. So the French didn't want any Black man coming to his country doing what I was doing. So the people said we going to buy it anyway and they couldn't stop me. Because a man who was paralyzed for 18 years named Filo Jean Lake—anyone 18 years old will remember he was in a wheel chair I took him out of that wheel chair. And when that spread to St. Martin Dr. Sebi became very, very, very, famous. I was very famous.

I agree with the Frenchmen when they put me in jail. Like I agree with the courts in New York when they put me in jail. In fact I sat and I told the attorney general that he was right to arrest me because I know that he couldn't fathom what I was doing, because no one before me had done so. I, myself, I'm just as equally amazed as everyone else around me because the amazement comes. I didn't put effort into acquiring what they say I know and what I've done.

Beverly: That's an interesting story but what about when you went to jail for trying to figure out what a plant was?

Dr. Sebi: I was trying to figure out the properties of the plant. I was in Brazil. I was in a place called Santos. There was a plant in the yard that I recognized and it was the condurango. I told Roosevelt I wanted to jump over there to see about the plant. The man called the cops. [DR. SEBI LAUGHS]

Beverly: The man who owned the property or Roosevelt?

Dr. Sebi: Roosevelt was my friend. He was telling Matun in New Orleans this. When I tell the story of herbology I begin in the 60s, late 60s. But Roosevelt said, "You crazy. Don't you remember when you nearly got us in trouble in Brazil because you saw that plant?" And that was in the 50s. So I was pursuing plants long before I even remember. Roosevelt told her that in New Orleans.

Beverly: So you jumped over into somebody's property, their yard?

Dr. Sebi: Yeah, I saw this plant. I saw this herb that attracted my attention and I knew the herb.

Beverly: Condurango? Did you pull it up?

Dr. Sebi: I didn't get time to get it. [WE LAUGH]

Beverly: What happened?

Dr. Sebi: The Brazilian man called the cops. Then they realized I was a foreigner and I told them that I knew the herbs because my parents used to use herbs.

Beverly: What did you think about doing with it?

Dr. Sebi: I don't know what I was going to do with it. I used to drink herbs way back then but not like I'm doing now.

Beverly: What did the police say when they arrived at that house in Brazil?

Dr. Sebi: At the house?

Beverly: Yes, when they came to pick you up.

Dr. Sebi: When the police came I was already leaving and they just came and asked us who are we. I said I was a merchant seaman, you know, a merchant seaman and I saw the plant.

Beverly: That is the 50s, right?

Dr. Sebi: Yeah.

Beverly: It never dawned on you during that time that you could make a medicine?

Dr. Sebi: Oh nah. I wasn't even interested in that. I was sick. I was sick in every form and fashion.

Beverly: It didn't dawn on you that what you were looking at in those yards and fields was something that could heal you?

Dr. Sebi: No. No. I had no idea that one day they would be part of my, very much a part of my journey.

Beverly: You get high off of healing and plants. Whenever you talk about the herbs and plants and nature, boy do you light up, get excited.

Dr. Sebi: "So, it's amazing. You didn't give energy to anything Dr. Sebi?" No. "Well how did you wind up with all this?" I don't know. Ask nature.

Beverly: The gods were with you.

Dr. Sebi: I never ask God for anything either.

Beverly: The Universe was with you whether you like it or know it or not.

Dr. Sebi: Yeah.

Beverly: It's Divine Order.

Dr. Sebi: Mama Hay told me that any man spends his life complementing woman, he's happy all his life. Any man that opposes women he's angry all his life. Well I chose the prior. I chose to be a slave to woman. And I love it because they love it too. And you know they can sense my acceptance of the totality of a woman. They take all kinds of privileges with me. They tell me all kinds of things.

Dr. Sebi drives around Usha Village and talks about future plans for the center. In addition to 14 huts, the sauna and bath houses, Usha Village has several structures for consultation and receiving visitors.

Dr. Sebi: I designed that kitchen and that dining room.

Beverly: It's beautiful.

Dr. Sebi: And he built it. The boy that's doing this built it. Look at the stars—in here, we are going to fill this up with sand because we are going to grow Love for a Moment right here. Love for a Moment is going to be in all of this.

Beverly: What is Love for a Moment?

Dr. Sebi: It's a beautiful plant, oh gosh, it's a beautiful flower. It looks like a rose but it's not. Then the water will be running in there. But the picket fence, where are we going to put the picket fence? Right here? Wait.

Beverly: Oh, there's a frog.

Dr. Sebi: Yeah. The picket will be here, in here. But that's a straight line. I like what he did. Beautiful.

Beverly: Love for a Moment. Where do you get that from?

Dr. Sebi: It grows here naturally. In the morning it's so pretty. Have you ever seen the red, red star in the morning?

Beverly: No.

Dr. Sebi: Well there's a little star I've been looking at ever since I was three years old. And I remember when I first saw that red star. I thought it was a candy. When you see it it's red, red, red, red. A red, red star.

Beverly: Listen to that water. That's beautiful.

Dr. Sebi: All this land is designated for agriculture, all of it. Also this is for agriculture. All of this would be for agriculture. This is for agriculture... If I move that from their baby [Matun] we could make a cluster of five beautiful huts right here, in that area. And it would be so pretty. But we are going to move that to here. And over here would be for the people of Honduras, right here. This would be the African Village that I'm talking about, second to none in the world. It's going to be right here. It's going to be pretty, clean, immaculate and functional.

Beverly: And your own garden and food, right here?

Dr. Sebi: We are growing everything that we eat.

Beverly: Okay. Oh, look at the ox.

Dr. Sebi: That's a bull.

Beverly: A bull?

Matun: Cattle.

Beverly: You've had this property for 20 years?

Dr. Sebi: Yep.

Beverly: You bought it from someone or is this part of your grandfather's property?

Dr. Sebi: No. My grandfather's property is in the islands. I bought this property. I bought it for $17,000.

Beverly: Oh my, all that? How many acres? That's a lot.

Dr. Sebi: About, how many acres? About 20.

Beverly: That's quite a bit. It looks like a lot.

Dr. Sebi: One of the things I give myself thanks for, and the only thing, is that I didn't let people come in and change the environment that I provided for myself or was provided for me. No, nobody penetrated that. I have had people to come and offer me millions of dollars to work with me, to do this, to take this internationally. I'm not impressed okay. I'm not impressed.

Beverly: You're satisfied with Usha, the Fig Tree, the company being on the level it is right now?

Dr. Sebi: No. I'm satisfied with me.

Beverly: You're happy.

Dr. Sebi: I always was. I always will be, until the day I die. It's easy. I don't consider myself strong or weak. I don't know what strong is or weak. I never lived that. You see, these are some of the things that most people don't know about Sebi. Sebi is not, was never poor and he will never be rich. Sebi, he doesn't know what strength is, no. He doesn't know what weakness is. He just lives. I just live. I don't know these things. I know I'm an individual that most people like and I'm an individual where there are some individuals that don't like me and both are right. They interpret me, they perceive me differently. So, about strength, I'm afraid of that word because, I consider myself a pussycat. I'm not a lion and that was told to me by a Korean girl named Kim that lived with us for about a year in Los Angeles. She noticed that when I talked, I talked with this lion voice. I have a great big voice.

Beverly: You have a strong voice.

Dr. Sebi: I have a strong voice. But she noticed that even though the strong voice come from me I'm a pussycat in behavior. And I laughed because she was right. I am a pussycat. And I like being a pussycat because the one thing that I never liked to know is that I injured someone in some way. I didn't want to do that. That I didn't want to do.

Agua Caliente—Usha Village

Beverly: What drove you to want to go back to La Ceiba.

Dr. Sebi: What drives me period, again, we try to find reason, "Well you know I did this and I did that." Yes, everything that you did was already predestined for you to do. This is why I never worry about anything, whether wife, whether money, whether healing, whether being a healer, whether losing it, whether anything. Because what's going to happen is going to happen anyway. And at 72 I'm thinking about going to Africa and build this thing for the Guinean people, when at 72, at 70, all my friends and brothers are dead. So why am I alive at 72 and talking about going to do something? Did I dictate that? No. That was dictated for me to do. Not that I was smart. Remember, I was the boy that didn't wear shoes until I was 13. So what did that have to do with anything? I still don't like shoes. But what does it have to do with the price of tea in China? Nothing whatsoever. I went to America from the position of Honduras, growing up in a forest. I met John Coltrane. I met Elijah Muhammad. I met Malcolm X. Look, I met a whole bunch of folks and I come out of the jungles of Honduras. But that was the journey I was supposed to make. Now I'm back in the jungle and boy do I like it better. I was telling my wife that I'm the king of the mountains. And why do I feel so good? These are the same mountains I saw as a little boy. But as a little boy I was wheezing with asthma. So I didn't enjoy life the way I would like to enjoy life because I was deprived of the very food that the body need to feed every cell, oxygen. So, my nerves were kind of shaky. But now I'm relaxed and I'm happy. I can enjoy the mountains, the same mountains with the clouds on them that I once walked across, the same river. I went to bathe in it the other day, just to feel it again.

Celebrities

Beverly: Stokely Carmichael.

Dr. Sebi: I met Stokely Carmichael many years, many, many, many years ago in New York, then Los Angeles.

Beverly: What was the experience like?

Dr. Sebi: 1972. I saw him again. Well, you know with me, what is the experience? I was in the car with Stokely Carmichael and Abbey Lincoln. And Stokely was talking about this revolutionary thing that he always talk about. This is what he knows. He knows about revolution. I prefer evolution. He was told, and I remember this distinctly, by Aminata [Abbey Lincoln], when he was talking weapons, she asked him, "Are guns the tools of our fathers?" And the boy looked stunned when Abbey Lincoln asked him that. "Are guns the tools of our fathers?" I know he couldn't answer that one. Because see, he wanted to change things. Well, I never wanted things to change. I want things to remain the way they are because that's the way they are supposed to be. If I want things to change do I know what they should change to? No. I don't have that dictated in my brain. He did. He was a Marxist. He was like Eldridge Cleaver. They were Marxists and revolutionists and Leninists. Me, I'm nothing. I was nothing. So I couldn't tell Mr. Stokely Carmichael anything that was worth anything to him. So I couldn't make any recommendations. But he came to me.

Beverly: He did?

Dr. Sebi: When his cancer was about to break loose and

Beverly: That was later on in life.

Dr. Sebi: Yes. He came to me and I gave him the compounds. And he began to urinate and he began to do well but he had to return to fight the revolution. And the food that revolutionary people eat is always hogs, starches and some uric acid.

Beverly: Lisa "Left Eye" Lopes, how did she come to see you?

Dr. Sebi: She was beautiful. She loved being Black. She loved knowing what she was doing and doing it. She loved life period. She was free. She used to walk from Beverly Hills and come and see me down in Venice, in Culver City. Lisa was balanced. Lisa had strength that I haven't seen in brothers who are males. Lisa knew that she was sick and that she wanted to be healed and that she wanted to get away from that place that she was in. And she did it. She came to me one night and she asked me what is it I'm supposed to do to get on the other side? I said fast as long as Jesus, 40 days and 40 nights. And she did it. And she told me that compassion was the only giving. Lisa Lopes, yes. I don't know if I'm really prepared to talk about Lisa the way that I would like to talk about her or the way that she is revealed to me. Because I find that in my life I have seen things and experienced things and it took me 20 years to fully understand what was happening for me to be able to talk about it. And Lisa Lopes is one of those persons that I know contributed a lot. Lisa Lopes contributed a lot to my existence. And Lisa Lopes helped me a lot in many ways emotionally. So Lisa, even though she was part of what you call the pop world, she could think. She was balanced. And she was compassionate and her intent with me was to unite with me. She was going to go to Africa with me. On the way back we would begin to develop the children's center, where children that are sick would come to the center and I would heal them. The design of the building died with her. And I couldn't tell her mother or brother what she had in mind because they build a square building there. I don't know for what.

Beverly: What was the first time you met Lisa?

Dr. Sebi: I don't remember the year, maybe 1996, 97.

Beverly: So you've had a relationship with her for a while.

Dr. Sebi: Um hum, 5 years.

Beverly: She came here to buy property.

Dr. Sebi: She bought the property right next to me.

Beverly: Is it still in her family?

Dr. Sebi: Sure. She bought it in my name.

Beverly: Michael Jackson. How did your relationship with Michael Jackson begin?

Dr. Sebi: The relationship with Michael Jackson begins the same way my relationship begins with Steven, with Ms. Cicely, with Teddy and everybody else that ever come to me. They come to me. So I was at home that Sunday afternoon.

Beverly: Home in Honduras?

Dr. Sebi: No. I was in Los Angeles with my wife and my daughter. And we were having a beautiful afternoon talking about the business we were going to do in Germany. Because I was invited to England and Germany and South America. So I'm still going to fulfill those...

Seven Days in Usha Village

Beverly: Obligations, invitations.

Dr. Sebi: Right. So here come Randy.

"Sebi! Sebi!" throwing rocks at the window.

So when I looked out I said that's Randy. What does he want now? Because I know that Randy is never serious. I knew that Randy wasn't a serious man about anything that is Black. How do I know that? Because Randy's been knowing me for years. Randy would bring his girlfriend to my house and they would sit in my bed and ask me all kinds of questions, never giving me the credit of knowing anything. Randy came and tell me that Michael wants to see me. I said for what? I wondered for what?

"What your brother want to see me for?"

"Well, he wants to see you."

I said okay. I'm going. When I get there Michael start talking. We went to Beverly Hills where his house is. He starts talking about this and that and the other, about he saw me in *Elle* magazine. That's what his secretary Grace Rwaramba said and a whole lot of other things. Well, it didn't make sense to me talking about he heard about me and this and that and the other. So I went back to my hotel, I mean to my office, my room. A week later they came back, Randy again.

"My brother wants you to travel with him."

Beverly: Where?

Dr. Sebi: I said fine. Just go talk about this. How much? I went to the house and they said they want me to travel with him, never saying that Michael is sick.

Celebrities

Now listen carefully. This indication was never made. You want me to travel with you. How much are you going to charge was the question.

I said, "I'm charging $4,000, uh $2,000 a day."

"Two thousand dollars a day?"

"Yes," I said, "or else I'll go back to my room and play with my wife and my baby. With me, it's very simple."

"Based on what?"

I said, "Eddie paid me $4,000 a day. I'm charging you half because I got to give you all of me. Traveling with you, it costs more than that because I'm being taken away from my business."

So he said okay. And I traveled. But when I went to Michael Jackson's house, I knew that whatever arrangement we had made wasn't going to be fulfilled. Because I saw a portrait of Michael in the sky in heaven with the white angels in his arms and the Black angels under his feet. So I knew that I wasn't going to receive the respect from Michael Jackson as did the other doctors that came to him and left him in a stupor that I had to take him out of. Because later on Ms. Grace Rwaramba would come to me and say Michael can't sleep. Michael is very nervous. Michael cannot sleep. Michael, Michael, Michael, Michael. I had to wake up all hours of the night to make special concoctions for Michael Jackson. This I did for five straight months. Then when I was not paid on the sixth I retreated. But I didn't expect for Michael to not pay me because his cooks became my patients. His cook's family became my patients. Jesus and the other one Rodolfo and Ann Hill.

They became my patients because they told me they didn't expect for him to recover.

Beverly: They didn't expect him to live?

Dr. Sebi: No.

Beverly: He was that sick?

Dr. Sebi: Yes. So Michael came back to life. When I submitted the bill, they reneged. Well, I could understand him reneging. That is understandable. My wife showed me repeatedly that I should not be angry at anyone knowing that they have been a recipient of glucose. It's as simple as that. But there's the law, which I had to revert to to get money from my brother for work that I have done. This is where we are at. I'm not surprised.

Beverly: Elizabeth Taylor.

Dr. Sebi: Well, she just donated money to UCLA to combat AIDS. But Elizabeth Taylor knows Michael Jackson because Michael Jackson called Elizabeth Taylor and told her about the diagnostic sheet that he, Michael Jackson saw, from laboratories and hospitals of people that were HIV positive who are no longer HIV positive. Elizabeth Taylor told Michael Jackson that my treatment should be free, but just a minute ago I look on television and Miss Elizabeth Taylor appears where she's donating money to UCLA to fight AIDS. But I'm supposed to give it away free. These are the things that exist in America that go unnoticed. Mr. Michael Jackson himself knows that I cure AIDS. But do you believe that he would take it upon himself to promote that? No. To think that is a dream. What we live is a nightmare.

Celebrities

Dr. Sebi allowed the printing of some of his clients' HIV diagnostic sheets. Since clinics and hospitals in Honduras performed the tests, all data is Spanish. But despite that, the terms "positivo" and "negativo" share the same meaning as English words "positive" and "negative" and they define a change in the patient's diagnosis. Three test sheets follow this section.

Dr. Sebi: Well, of all the celebrities that I have treated or their families, the one that make me feel like a human being and that I deserve to be alive, one and only one, him, his mother, his brother Charlie and his uncle Charlie, and everybody in his house—Eddie Murphy. Yes, I could vouch for Eddie Murphy as being one of the most sane individuals that I interrelated with, and considerate.

HOSPITAL VICENTE D'ANTONI

DEPARTAMENTO DE LABORATORIO Y BANCO DE SANGRE

Nombre _____ *Zavala.* _____ No. Hospital _____

Dr. _____ Clave _____

EXAMEN DE:

H. I.V = Positivo

FECHA 25 /NOV. 93 _____ FIRMA _____

Copia

Patient Zavala's Test Results
November 25, 1993 (Positive)

HOSPITAL VICENTE D'ANTONI

DEPARTAMENTO DE LABORATORIO Y BANCO DE SANGRE

Nombre _____ *Zavala.* _____ No. Hospital _____

Dr. _____ Clave _____

EXAMEN DE:

H.I.V = NEGATIVO

FECHA _13/enero 94_ FIRMA _____

copia

Patient Zavala's Test Results
January 13, 1994 (Negative)

SEROLOGIA

PRUEBA	RESULTADO
ELISA-HIV	POSITIVO
HBs Ag (Hepatitis B)	////////
T. cruzi (Chagas)	////////
R. P. R.	////////

Nota: LO ANTERIOR REFIERE QUE SE HAGA LA PRUEBA CONFIRMATORIA
DE WESTERN BLOT.

Patient Josue's Test Results, 1994 (Positive)

102

LIC. LIZETH PA
Jefe de Laboratorio

Laboratorio Paredes
ANALISIS CLINICOS

Clínicas Andrade	10 Calle entre Ave. San
Ave. Morazán Sur 92	Isidro y la República
Tels. 43-09-93	49-0366	Tel. 43-02-90
La Ceiba, Honduras, C. A.	

NOMBRE __JOsue__

MEDICO _____

FECHA __19 de enero de 1995__

Tip. Moderna RTN-9EQYPP-3 6-94 20

MUESTRA   De Sangre

H.I.V......: Negative

Patient Josue's Test Results, January 19, 1995 (Negative)

103

Laboratorio Paredes
ANALISIS CLINICOS

Clínicas Andrade · 10 Calle entre Ave. San
Ave. Morazán Sur 92 · Ictaro y la República
Tels. 43-00-03 / 43-0368 · Tel. 43-02-90
La Ceiba, Honduras, C. A.

NOMBRE ———— Suárez

MEDICO ————

FECHA ———— 2 de agosto de 1994

T.p. Moderna RTN-9BQYPP-3 6-84

MUESTRA de sangre

H.I.V. .... Positivo

FIRMA ————

Patient Suarez's Test Results, August 2, 1994 (Positive)

Laboratorio Paredes
ANALISIS CLINICOS

Clínicas Andrade | 10 Calle entre Ave. San
Ave. Morazán Sur 92 | Isidro y la República
Tels. 43-09-23 | 43-0368   Tel. 43-02-90
La Ceiba, Honduras, C. A.

NOMBRE————————————————
MEDICO————————————————
FECHA———— 19 de Agosto de 1994

T:p. Moderna RTN-9EQYPP-3 6-94

MUESTRA De Sangre

H.I.V...........:Negativo

FIRMA————————————————

Patient Suarez's Test Results, August 19, 1994 (Negative)

105

EPILOGUE

Beverly: If people are inspired by the book does it matter?

Dr. Sebi: Some, there may be thousands who may be inspired. And there may be millions that disagree. That doesn't matter with me. My mother told me that the only reason I should write the book, not because I told her, but I say, "Mother, you heard the public ask me on numerous times where is your book?" Well, if I write a book this is another book on the shelf, just another book on the shelf. Because people read books and after they read them they put them on the shelf and they gather dust. Well, I don't have any books in my house. "And mother, since I never read a book in my life and I do not have any books in my house, why should I write this?" "Because it is not your book. It is your observation of nature and what you have benefit from your observation against others who have said they have observed nature too. But they haven't done what you have done." You see. So her answer was you are going to show them what nature is saying, that we have disobeyed because we didn't know.

Beverly: I agree with your mother.

Dr. Sebi: Well my mother has never given me an answer that was inequitable. My mother has given me every answer. My mother and my grandmother gave me was right on time. If it wasn't on time I would not have reached this level of expression because I know that all through my life what my mother and my grandmother share with their son, Sebi, I used. And I never got myself in trouble with anyone or anything. People got themselves in trouble with me, like the law. The law said arrest this man because he's lying. But that is America. America have to say I'm lying. Have they ever heard of such of thing? Furthermore, in America people always ask you which is a bit of an insult to us, when you guys

107

come here and do that—you all say, "Is that true?" Oh my God, we walk away because you telling me I'm lying. But in America it is customary to ask someone, after they have said something, "Is that true?" Look, that's an insult. That's really, really, really out. But it is not an insult in America. Because when the attorney general arrested me he said I was a charlatan. Now what is a charlatan? A liar. Now why did he creep into his brain and imagine that? Because he lives a lie. You could only think of someone lying if you're a liar because if you live clean and live truth you never would entertain that someone else is lying, never.

Cosmic Arrangement

Dr. Sebi: So we are never satisfied with the things of the moment that we are given. Like for instance, I asked the question, slavery, was it supposed to occur?

Beverly: Are you asking me?

Dr. Sebi: Yes.

Beverly: Uh,

Dr. Sebi: Well how did it occur?

Beverly: The Europeans came in?

Dr. Sebi: Because, because, because, but then, did it occur?

Beverly: It did occur.

Dr. Sebi: Okay. So that's the reality. Now that we know that we came and they brought us from Africa, where in Africa would you like to go to and live right now or you identify with? You don't know. Nobody knows. We know that we are living this experience we call America. Understand? That is the reality, whether we want to or not. But if we stop and we accept the reality that this is it regardless to what this is, we live it gracefully and then we enjoy it because that is what it is. We're not in Africa no longer. And by the way I want to say this, in my journey from there to here, from my inception, from my birth to this age of 72, the one thing that I always steadfast held to was the essence of Africa, the basic ingredients of Africa. And how was I able to extrapolate from Africa these basic ingredients or principles? Well, it was easy for me, there again. Like curing AIDS is easy. I notice that the African people didn't leave Africa to go and conquer the land of another. The African people didn't enslave another. So these things tell me that my ancestors afforded the one thing that the world needs most today, love and compassion. And to see that I, Dr. Sebi, cling to those two little things knowing that we are nonoffensive. We're not warriors. Brothers and sisters today who have a late history of Africa like to say that we were warriors. We were generals. We were all of these things. We were never any of that. We were peaceful people living in the forest without any clothes on. We didn't have any hospitals. We didn't have any doctors. We didn't have any rapes. We didn't have any delinquency. We just lived as God designed us to live. It's as simple as that.

Beverly: That's the reality.

Dr. Sebi: Yes. So the message is here. Black people are not supposed to put blood in their mouth. Why? Because it confounds things. Now, example, when I say confounds things, it prevents you from seeing. I was given a disease that I had to address, a disease that you would never find the solution in any book. That disease is known as lockjaw.

109

Beverly: Lockjaw?

Dr. Sebi: Lockjaw. Once your jaw is locked it will remain locked and you will die. So I sit in front of her and I saw her dying and everybody was in the house, approximately 100 people. And it come to my skull. You call yourself a healer. Now this woman is dying. You know you can't go to any books because there aren't any books that have within the pages, its pages, the answer to lockjaw. So you better go into yourself. And what did I come up with? What I came up with, I came up with the answer from within me. The answer was to go to her skull. And I went to her skull. And I went to her skull because her jaw was locked, meaning that the organ that is responsible for her jaw being locked is her brain. I cannot go through her mouth like I usually do to give someone a substance. The mouth is locked. So I have to go where? The nearest point to her brain—her skull— because her skull is porous. The same herb that I would have given her in her mouth, I put it on her skull wet, hot. And she opened her mouth in 15 minutes or less. So where do you go and find that information? It comes from us but we are not trusting in ourselves and the reason why we do not trust ourselves is because we don't even trust God. When we stop trusting God, we stop trusting self. Because look, correct me if I'm wrong. Every book on the planet, whether the Bhagavad-Gita, the Talmud, the Torah or the Koran and not to mention the Holy Bible, it is stated that the herbs are for the healing of the Nation. But the followers of these religions, when they get sick, where do they go? To the herbs or to a chemical? Well, we don't want to go further because it's embarrassing. So as we look at this picture, seeing that the very substance, one of the components that should not be overlooked, which is our health and the medicine of our body, we tell God to go to hell, literally.

Beverly: Because we take drugs?

Dr. Sebi: Because they gave us sugar. The hypothalamus gland has been interfered with. It cannot process anymore. It cannot decipher. It cannot help you. It has turned against you. But as soon as we abstain from the things that program the hypothalamus gland—clarity, like in the case of my wife dying, and I went to her skull, who helped me to go there? I did because my brain was clear enough. And if all of us was to go there you wouldn't need Sebi. We would all be seeing. But right now I'm a one-eyed man where everybody is blind. Well, one-eyed man is king where everybody is blind. But I only have one eye open. This is serious. It's very serious. But as we look at the full picture now we see that all of the conversations and all of the dialogue and the meetings were based solely on that confused hypothalamus gland. That's why the result is not seeing, like my wife was showing you.

Because like I said when I went to Zimbabwe and I showed these people with diagnostic sheets from laboratories that they support, and they rejected it, I knew they were disrespectful. And that is all I needed to see. That's all I needed to see. I'm not going to make any excuses for Africa. No. There's only one country in Africa that I would return to and that's the country of Guinea. No other. And I mean no other. Because my word is bond and bond is life. And I give my life before my word prevail. I will go to one if I'm forcibly taken to one, not of my own volition. I will never return to South Africa. I'm going to mention them. South Africa, Zimbabwe, Tanzania, Nigeria; never will I return to them and all the West African countries, except Guinea. Why? Because they, the African people that I mentioned, they blatantly disrespected the entity. They also make very fun of me, which I like and I agree. I loved it because it tells me about their conscience and their compassion. It tells me where they are at. Yet they tell the world that

111

they would do anything to combat the ravages of AIDS. That is far from the truth. There isn't any African country in Africa but one that is interested in the eradication of AIDS or any other disease—Guinea. No other country is interested in that. How I know? Because they know about me and they know I cure AIDS. It's as simple as that, common sense.

Beverly: What have those countries done to you?

Dr. Sebi: What have they done? They just said to hell with you. It's as simple as that, or get out of here. Some even said f#%k you, straight out f#%k. [DR. SEBI SPELLS IT OUT] I don't want to mention the country, right? But plain old f#%k you. I said thank you sir. Oh I was happy. I was happy because maybe that's what I was going to do that night. [HE LAUGHS SARCASTICALLY] I didn't care. So I know what exists on this planet as far as compassion and consciousness and giving, no, that doesn't exist. Ethics and morality do not exist. It never existed. Those are words. But the act does not exist. The state does not exist. They're words, ethical, moral. Sounds good.

Beverly: I'm still trying to get a picture of this foundation. Is there anything else Mama Hay said besides walk naked if you find yourself without provisions?

Dr. Sebi: That was sufficient. I interpreted it in a way that she wanted me to receive it, you see. But in America that's arrogance because that's how they perceive me, as arrogant, when I talk the way I talk. In fact, it was recently my mother told me when she looked at the tape when I was speaking in Washington, I was very angry at the audience. And she told me that I was the only angry person there. But she understood why I was angry. I was dissatisfied because why should I have a piece of information and no one else in the community has that information. That doesn't put me in a good position. It put me in a vulnerable position. Because it tells me how weak we are, how vulnerable the whole race really is. Because in the forest what one gorilla knows, all gorillas know. What one Black man in the forest knows, every Black man knew. Not now. Because I didn't go to grade school. He went to grade school. The other one went to high school. They all went to the BS. The other one masters degree and then the doctorate degree. So now when we put all these degrees into the sequence of life, we find that the degrees will undermine the carrier of it and those that are less fortunate because he uses it against them. But in the forest there were no degrees. Everybody was on the same plane. But the man with the degree thought he spent his time acquiring the degree to get wisdom for what? No. The wisdom or the knowledge he acquired was to produce in an industry. It wasn't to enhance his life. That was the mistake that was made. The doctorate degree doesn't guarantee your health nor your happiness. It guarantees you making more money to buy more things to damage your body even more. But it doesn't guarantee happiness. But the one that doesn't have the degree, he's offended by the one that has the degree because he would like to have had that doctorate degree. Well with me, it was a little bit different. I didn't need the degree. I didn't want the degree because if I had received a degree from someone, then it would have gone against the grain of my grandmother.

Beverly: Would you like to go back to those Weather Report days, John Coltrane days? Were we better off then?

Dr. Sebi: I never use the word better. That is never in my vocabulary.

Seven Days in Usha Village

Beverly: The quality of life, it was different.

Dr. Sebi: It was happy. I know it was very happy but it's happy now because, see, I have left that age group. If you talk to the age group now that I was in in the days of 'Trane and Little Richard and all those people, I'm going to tell you that I was happy because I was in my 20s. So when you talk to someone in their 20s now, with pop, they happy too because they don't want to know about politics and all that stuff. I didn't know about politics and all that stuff. We were happy. We were doing it. So therefore were they better days? For who? For me? No, because right now I'm living my better days. When I was in New Orleans I had asthma. I haven't had asthma in 42 years. So my better days are now, where I'm enjoying my life. I'm enjoying my life but it is on the same level of quality as it was when I was in my 20s because I at least had more energy to exert. But I remember having to breathe very heavy sometimes, many times, many, many times. But the people were happy and the girls were happy. It didn't take too much to take a girl out. You could go out with two dollars and you buy your tickets for a dollar and you still had change. You could buy a hamburger for 15 cents or 20 cents, 25 cents, and a malt for 15 cents. And the ticket's a quarter. So you see, you have a lot of money left. And it was easy. We didn't have crack. But now to take your girlfriend out you better ask her, "Hey girl what do you get down with? What's your preference of drugs? I know you have one. You must be taking drugs. What is it?" So, it has changed a little, right? But I know that those things are seemingly difficult. You'd be surprised how they could shift. Overnight they could shift. But as human beings always used to show me, we are more intelligent than animals. And because we are more intelligent than animals, well, I know that it doesn't take much for human beings to listen to something and realize that it

EPILOGUE

has value. Gorillas, they don't have to listen to another gorilla because what one gorilla knows, all gorillas know.

GLOSSARY

A

acid plants—plants having a pH of less than 7

Afrika, Dr. Llaila—Black American herbalist, author of *African Holistic Health*

Aguan River—in northern Honduras, 150 miles long, from central highlands west of Yoro down to the Caribbean Sea

Airola, Paavo—(1918-1983) nutritionist, naturopathic physician and author of numerous books on natural healing, including *How to Get Well: Handbook of Natural Healing*

alkaline—having a pH greater than 7; containing alkali

amaranth—natural grain, annuals having dense clusters of tiny flowers

apartheid—former policy of racial segregation practiced in the Republic of South Africa

Aristotle—(384-322 B.C.) Greek philosopher

ayurvedic—traditional Hindu system of medicine based on homeopathy and naturopathy

B

Belize—Central American country on the Caribbean Sea

Bethune, Mary McLeod—(1875-1955) Black American educator, founder of the Daytona Normal and Industrial Institute, which, in 1923, became Bethune-Cookman College

Bhagavad-Gita—(India c. 500 B.C.) means "song of the Lord," a classic writing of Indian spirituality

biochemically—relating to chemical substances and vital processes in living organisms

Bishop Noel Jones—(1950-) pastor of the City of Refuge Church in Los Angeles

117

B

blue vervain—perennial herb, edible and medicinal, short leaf stalks, flowers are pale lilac and 5-petaled; used as an antidiarrheal, analgesic, astringent, sedative; useful for ulcers, rheumatism and colds

bovine—ox, cow

bromides—compounds with bromine in a formal oxidation state of –1; as potassium bromide, frequently used as a sedative in the late 19th and early 20th century

Brynner, Yul—(1915-1985) leading actor in American films, director

burdock—weedy plant with purplish flowers surrounded by prickly bracts and forming a bur in fruit

Butts, Reverend Calvin—(1949-) pastor of the historic Abyssinian Baptist Church in Harlem, New York

C

carbonic acid—a weak dibasic acid formed when carbon dioxide dissolves in water; it forms carbonate and bicarbonate

Carmichael, Stokely—aka Kwame Toure (1941-1998) Black social activist born in Trinidad, graduate of Howard University, field organizer, then chairman of the Student Nonviolent Coordinating Committee (SNCC)

carnivorous—carnivore, flesh-eating

cassava—perennial woody shrub, grown as an annual; tropical root crop grown for its enlarged starch-filled roots

cellular (cell)—the smallest unit of life that carries out its own processes (organelles); organelles allow the cell to function properly

charlatan—quack, medical fraud

collard greens—various loose-leafed cultivars of the cabbage plant; the plant is grown for its large, dark-colored edible leaves; classified in same cultivar group as kale and spring greens

C

Coltrane, John—(1926-1967) Black American jazz musician; avant-garde tenor saxophonist

commissary—a store for provisions, food supplies, usually on military bases

Community Warehouse—former Washington, DC-based health food co-op and cultural center for art, music and lectures

condurango—bark of a South American vine of the milkweed family

Cooke, Sam—(1931-1964) Black American gospel, rhythm and blues, and pop singer, composer

cosmic—powerful energies of unknown quantity perceived by humans through direct observation, meditation/contemplation

cyanide—any of various compounds containing a CN group, especially poisonous compounds potassium cyanide and sodium cyanide

D

Daddy Grace—aka Charles M. Daddy (1881-1960) founder of the United House of Prayer

Dalai Lama—(1935-) Buddhist priest; 14th Dalai Lama of Tibet

dandelion—a weedy plant having many-rayed yellow flower heads; juice of the root, bitter and milky, used for medicinal purposes

Diogenes—(404-323 B.C.) Cynic philosopher from Sinope (a city of Turkey on the Black Sea)

dong quai—herb used in traditional Chinese medicine, blooming clusters of white flowers

E

echinacea—purple coneflower herb used for stimulating the immune system and treating infectious diseases

Elle **Magazine**—worldwide magazine that focuses on women's fashion, beauty, health and entertainment

Ellington, Duke—(1899-1974) Black American jazz musician, composer and band leader

F
Farrakhan, Louis—(1933-) Black American Muslim leader of the Nation of Islam, former Calypso singer

Father Divine—(1880-1965) Black American religious leader and founder of the International Peace Mission Movement

fonio—a small cultivated natural grain or millet used in cereals, porridge, bread and couscous; crops found in Savannas of West Africa

G
gari—made from cassava, which is grated and the excess liquid is squeezed out; remaining cassava is then fried over an open fire on a broad metal pan

Garvey, Marcus—(1887-1940) Black nationalist, born in Jamaica, founder of the Universal Negro Improvement Association

glucose—a monosaccharide sugar that occurs widely in most plant and animal tissue and is the major energy source of the body

guru—a personal spiritual teacher; revered teacher or mentor

H
Hamilton, Roy—(1929-1969) Black American R&B and pop singer in the 1950s

herbivorous—plant eating

Homo sapiens—the modern species of humans

hybrid—offspring of genetically dissimilar species; mixed composition

hypothalamus—the part of the brain that lies below the thalamus and regulates bodily temperature, certain metabolic processes and other autonomic activities

I
iodides—a binary compound of iodine usually with a more electro-positive element or radical

iron—pure silver-white element, when chemically active, plays a vital role in biological processes as in transporting oxygen in the body

K
Kaposi's sarcoma—a cancer characterized by bluish-red nodules on the skin

K
Koran or Quran—the sacred text of Islam, considered by Muslims to contain the revelations of God to Muhammad

L
lactic acid—a syrupy liquid present in sour milk, molasses and various fruits

Lincoln, Abbey—aka Aminata (1930-) Black American jazz vocalist, songwriter and actress

Little Richard—(1932-) Black American rock and roll singer and piano player

lockjaw—infection that causes extreme muscle stiffness and spasms; caused by the germ *clostridium tetani* that enters body through a puncture wound

M
macrobiotic—practice of promoting well-being and longevity, especially by means of a diet chiefly of whole grains and beans

Mahdi—Islamic messiah expected to appear at the world's end and establish peace

Malcolm X—aka El Hajj Malik El-Shabazz (1925-1965) Black American Muslim Minister and speaker for the Nation of Islam

Mudsimi Wakanaka—a food preparation component of Dr. Sebi's Office, LLC

Muhammad, Elijah—(1897-1975) Black American nationalist and leader of the Nation of Islam

N
neuropathology—the study of disease of the nervous system

Noble Drew Ali—(1886-1929) Black American religious leader and founder of the Moorish Science Temple of America

O
oxalic acid—a poisonous strong acid that occurs in various plants as oxalates

P
pH—a measure of the acidity or alkalinity of a plant or solution

pH scale—barometer used to measure how acidic or alkaline a substance is; the pH scale ranges from 0 to

14; a pH of 7 is neutral; a pH less than 7 is acidic while a pH greater than 7 is alkaline

P
phosphorous—a highly reactive, nonmetallic element

Plato—(428-347 B.C.) Greek philosopher

Platters, The—American vocal group of the 1950s rock & roll era

potassium phosphate—one of three orthophosphates of potassium

Q
quinoa—natural grain, a pigweed of the high Andes of South America widely used as a cereal in Peru

S
sea moss—seaweed, various red algae from rose to violet

septic—causing sepsis, which is the presence of pathogenic organisms or their toxins in the blood or tissues

Shook, Edward—renowned herbalist and author of *Advanced Treatise in Herbology*

Socrates—(469-399 B.C.) Greek philosopher

spelt—a nutritious and ancient grain with a nutty flavor, type of wheat

sulfur—essential element for life; abundant, tasteless multivalent nonmetal; yellow crystalline solid in its native form; in nature, a pure element or as sulfide and sulfate minerals

T
Talmud—the collection of ancient Rabbinic writings constituting the basis of religious authority in Orthodox Judaism

Tata tonic—liquid herbal energizer manufactured by Dr. Sebi's Office, Inc.

teff—an economically important African cereal grass used for its grain, which yields a forage and hay crop

thermal—using, producing, or caused by heat

Torah—first five books of the Hebrew scriptures

Tubman, Harriet—(1820-1913) Black American abolitionist, former slave and leader in the Underground Railroad

U
UCLA—University of California, Los Angeles

uric acid—a semisolid compound that is the chief nitrogenous component of the urine in birds and reptiles

V
Vaughan, Sara—(1924-1990) Black American jazz singer

Y
yellow dock—a short-lived perennial herb commonly used as a laxative in cases of maldigestion and low stomach acid

NOTE

The natural grains Dr. Sebi mentioned—spelt, quinoa, amaranth—can be found in major health and natural food stores in the form of cereals, flour, pastas, dinner rolls, and loaves of bread.

Made in United States
Troutdale, OR
04/28/2024

19503839R00080